Good Fats for Women's Health Cookbook

Delicious Recipes for Menopausal Balance

Dr. Olivia Tastewell

Disclaimer: The information in this book is intended as general guidance and education. It should not be used as a substitute for medical advice from your doctor or qualified health professional about your specific situation. The author and publisher expressly disclaim any liability, loss, or risk incurred, directly or indirectly, as a result of the use of any of the contents of this book.

Table of Contents

SIMPLE EXERCISES AND SELF-CARE PRACTICES FOR MENOPAUSE .. 119

CONCLUSION **123**

INTRODUCTION

As the warm summer breeze rustles the wind chimes on my patio, I sink back into the cushioned chair with a sigh. My once energetic 53-year-old self feels like a distant memory as another wave of fatigue washes over me. This relentless exhaustion seems to have settled into my very bones ever since those first hot flashes and night sweats started disrupting my sleep a couple years ago.

My experience is distressingly common for the millions of women who find themselves squarely in the throes of menopause each year. This natural biological transition, marking the end of a woman's reproductive years, typically begins in the 40s or 50s. It's initiated by a gradual decline in reproductive hormones like estrogen and progesterone, triggering an onslaught of uncomfortable physical and emotional changes that can upend a woman's normal quality of life.

Overview of Menopause and Common

Symptoms

I was wholly unprepared for the vast array of symptoms menopause can bring on over the course of its multiple stage progression. For most women, the first signs are irregular periods and those telltale hot flashes - sudden feelings of intense heat, sweating, and flushing that can last for several minutes. Many of us also struggle with night sweats, leaving our beds drenched in perspiration even as winter temperatures plummet.

As hormone levels continue shifting, a constellation of other symptoms often arises. Brain fog and forgetfulness become frequent frustrations, along with distracting bouts of anxiety or unexplained mood changes. Flagging energy makes it difficult to tackle basic tasks, compounded by disrupted sleep from insomnia or those nagging night sweats. While I had heard about hot flashes, I wasn't expecting this profound, full-body fatigue.

One of the most discouraging aspects of menopause can be the unwanted weight gain that tends to occur, particularly around the abdomen. Despite eating the same healthy diet, I've watched in dismay as the numbers on the scale keep creeping upward and my once well-fitting pants grow snugger. This weight gain results from hormonal impacts on metabolism as well as how fat becomes distributed in the body.

Joint aches, headaches, breast tenderness, skin irritation, and a host of other symptoms are also par for the course. Every woman's experience with the timing and severity of these changes is quite unique. What we all have in common is the struggle to feel like our normal, vital selves as our bodies take us through the climacteric years leading up to menopause.

The Importance of Healthy Fats for

Menopausal Health

While there's no way to completely circumvent the roller coaster of menopause, focusing on diet and lifestyle adjustments can make a world of difference in minimizing those debilitating symptoms. This is where the importance of incorporating more healthy fats into your meals simply cannot be overstated.

The right balance of dietary fats is absolutely crucial during menopause for optimal hormone production and overall physical and mental well-being. Despite being perfectly healthy eaters for decades, many women unknowingly drop their intake of good fats too low as they transition into menopause. At a time when consuming fats from high-quality sources is more vital than ever, our diets are falling short.

That's because the body relies on healthy fats to manufacture hormones like estrogen in the years after the ovaries become inactive. Omega-3 fatty acids from fish, walnuts, and seeds are particularly critical for promoting balanced hormones and reducing the intensity of hot flashes, night sweats, and mood disturbances. Monounsaturated fats from olive oil, avocados, and nuts help enable fat-burning and weight control while offsetting the metabolic slowdown of menopause.

There's also mounting research connecting healthy fats to protection against some of the elevated disease risks of menopause. They help optimize cholesterol levels to guard against heart disease. Certain fatty acids are linked to reducing breast cancer risk and cognitive decline. By delivering fat-soluble vitamins like A, D, E and K, healthy fats provide potent antioxidants for anti-aging benefits.

In essence, getting ample amounts of the right dietary fats helps smooth the hormonal transition of menopause while preventing weight gain, fatigue, and inflammation - the root causes of so many of my menopause symptoms. These healthy fats are essentially a menopausal woman's best friend and closest ally as her body pushes through this change of life.

How This Cookbook Can Help

But for me and countless other women, knowing which fats to prioritize and how to incorporate them into daily life is utterly befuddling. That's where this cookbook comes to the rescue as your comprehensive guide to harnessing the powers of healthy fats.

These pages are brimming with more than 100 easy, delicious recipes that highlight the top sources of nourishing dietary fats like salmon, avocados, olive oil, nuts, and seeds. Whether I'm rushed in the morning or entertaining friends, I'll find crave-worthy options for breakfasts, lunches, dinners, snacks, and even decadent treats. And I can feel good about enjoying every single bite, because they've been carefully crafted by nutritionists to deliver the satisfying flavors and textures, I crave without sending my hormones into a tailspin.

But this book has so much more to offer than just recipes alone. Before we dive into the delectable dishes, you'll gain a thorough understanding of the types of fats to embrace and avoid for menopausal health, along with specifics on how they can ease symptoms like hot flashes, insomnia, weight fluctuations, and more. We'll explore the top food sources for omega-3s, monounsaturated fats, and other nutrients that promote balanced hormones and cardiovascular vitality.

You'll also find helpful tips for setting up your kitchen for healthy menopause eating success. Learn savvy shopping strategies, meal prepping advice, healthier substitutions for cutting calories and added sugars, and simple culinary hacks for maximum flavor. Plus, you'll have access to printable tools like trackable meal plans and symptom journals to help you stay motivated and connected to your wellness goals.

This cookbook recognizes that menopause is as much an emotional journey as a physical one. That's why you'll find uplifting stories woven throughout from real women who have traversed the menopause transition themselves. Their hard-won wisdom and glimpses into relatable struggles provide empowering reminders that you've got this - and that food can be a powerful source of comfort and nourishment as you navigate this often-rocky terrain.

By focusing my diet around luscious, health-promoting fats, I'll be giving my body the nutrient foundation it needs to minimize menopause symptoms while protecting against long-term health impacts. These recipes allow me to savor each forkful knowing it's delivering vitality rather than hormonal havoc. This book is my gateway to rediscovering the energy, balanced moods, clear thinking and overall vibrancy I thought might be lost forever.

So, let's raise a fork to reclaiming control and joie de vivre during this transition. With the power of good fats fueling me through menopause, the hot flashes, fatigue, and muffin top will no longer define this remarkable chapter of life. It's time to feel like my best self again!

Chapter 1: The Power of Good Fats

When my hot flashes first kicked into high gear, leaving me flushed and drenched in sweat, I desperately searched for solutions. I tried breathing exercises, dressing in lightweight layers, even turning my home into a frosty cave with the air conditioning. But nothing could tame those searing sensations of heat that would wash over me at any given moment.

Little did I know that one of the most effective natural remedies for easing my hormonal woes was sitting right there in my kitchen pantry and fridge - healthy dietary fats. Yes, the very fats I had been avoiding for years in an attempt to stay slim and trim actually possess incredible powers when it comes to managing menopause symptoms from the inside out.

You see, our bodies absolutely need fats in optimal amounts to function properly at every stage of life. But during that pivotal transition into menopause, consuming the right kinds of fats becomes crucial for smoothing hormonal ups and downs while combating those aggravating side effects like hot flashes, weight creep, and fatigue. Not only that, but prioritizing good fats can help protect our hearts, bones, and brains too.

The truth is, fat has gotten an unjustly bad reputation for far too long - something I bought into hook, line and sinker as a young woman. By better understanding the different types of fats and how they can nurture our bodies through the menopausal change, we can finally embrace their role in feeling and looking our best as we navigate this new stage of life.

Types of Healthy Dietary Fats

Let's start by clearing up any lingering confusion around dietary fats so we're all on the same page. We need three main varieties in our diets - monounsaturated fats, polyunsaturated fats, and a type of polyunsaturated called omega-3 fatty acids. In simple terms, these are the "good" fats we want to make room for.

Monounsaturated fats can help lower bad LDL cholesterol levels while raising good HDL cholesterol. They're typically liquid at room temperature but start to solidify when chilled. Some of the best sources are olive oil, olives, avocados, almonds, cashews, peanuts, and peanut butter.

Then we have polyunsaturated fats, deemed "healthy" because they're a crucial building block for our cells and assist the body with critical functions like blood clotting, muscle movement, and regulating inflammation. You'll find them in abundance in sunflower, corn, soybean, and vegetable oils as well as walnuts, pine nuts, and sesame seeds.

Omega-3 fatty acids are a star subset of polyunsaturated fats because our bodies can't produce them on their own - we have to get them from the foods we eat. There are three main types: ALA from plant sources like chia, flax, and walnuts, and then EPA and DHA predominantly found in fatty fish like salmon, mackerel, and sardines.

Therefore, in review, we've got our monounsaturated fats from plants and plant-based oils, our polyunsaturated fats also from plants and plant oils, and then those coveted omega-3 fatty acids from both plants and fatty fish. Getting the right balance of all three is essential.

By contrast, the two types of fats we want to minimize or avoid completely are saturated fats and trans fats.

Saturated fats from fried foods, fatty meats, butter, and the like can raise our LDL or "bad" cholesterol levels when eaten in excess. And trans fats, created through an industrial process of hydrogenation, have been shown to increase disease risk even in small amounts.

Now that we've got a better handle on fat basics, let's dive into why those "good" fats are so powerful for managing menopause.

Benefits of Good Fats for Menopause

Ever since my oncologist broke the bad news that I was officially going through "the change," I've felt like my body has been a ticking time bomb waiting to go off. One minute, I'm sleeping like a baby. The next, I'm jolting awake in a puddle of sweat from night sweats. In the morning, my energy banks are totally tapped out before my feet even hit the floor. And don't even get me started on this thickening waistline!

But focusing on getting those high-quality dietary fats into my daily routine has been a total gamechanger for taming my most disruptive menopause symptoms. By being more mindful about including foods like avocados, olive oil, nuts, seeds, and fatty fish at mealtimes, I've experienced significant relief and a renewed sense of balance.

First off, healthy fats like the omega-3s from seafood can be our BFFs when it comes to fighting those dreaded hot flashes. They help regulate reproductive hormones like estrogen, progesterone, and testosterone, minimizing the intensity and frequency of night sweats too. Not having to constantly rip off layers or keep a towel draped over my pillow? Yes, please!

These good fats are also total MVPs when it comes to combating insomnia and fatigue. Omega-3s have been clinically shown to improve sleep quality by increasing melatonin production and reducing inflammation. Fats like those in avocados, olive oil, and nuts promote sharper focus and steadier energy levels by helping our bodies use glucose and protein for fuel more efficiently.

As if that wasn't enough, healthy fats can be potent weight loss allies in our fight against that dreaded muffin top or meno-pot. By eating more good fats at meals and snacks, they trigger a molecular "switch" that signals our bodies to stop storing fat and start burning it for energy instead. Fats also keep us feeling fuller for longer so we're not as tempted by those late-night snack cravings that sabotage our best efforts.

Furthermore, maintaining a diet rich in monounsaturated and polyunsaturated fats has been shown to lower risks for some of the most concerning health issues associated with menopause, like heart disease, osteoporosis, breast cancer, and cognitive decline. The omega-3s in fish are particularly potent for optimizing cholesterol levels and reducing inflammation, a driving force behind so many chronic illnesses.

Let's not forget how fats contribute to healthy, glowing skin and hair during a life stage notorious for those areas showing signs of aging and thinning. Good fats are loaded with antioxidant vitamins like A, D, E, and K, renowned for protecting our bodies from oxidative stress and free radical damage. Some studies have even suggested omega-3s can preserve collagen, that essential protein that keeps complexions smooth and plump.

I know firsthand how quickly a hot flash or night sweat can crush your self-confidence when you're in the throes of this hormonal rollercoaster. But keeping my body well-stocked with quality fats has done wonders for taming menopausal chaos from the inside out. I'm no longer a slave to my symptoms or feeling like a shell of my former self.

With the right fats in your nutritional cornerstone, you too can start reclaiming your vitality and a sense of control during this unpredictable phase of womanhood. This transformation won't happen overnight, but consistently nurturing your body with these health-promoting nutrients can smooth the bumps in your menopausal journey. Next up, we'll discover the very best food sources to stock your kitchen with!

Unhealthy fats to limit (trans fats, fried foods)

By now, I hope you're feeling inspired to embrace more of those health-boosting monounsaturated, polyunsaturated and omega-3 fatty acids into your daily routine. But just as important as increasing the good fats is being aware of which ones to strictly limit or avoid altogether during this delicate menopausal season.

You see, not all fats are created equal in terms of their impact on our hormones, hearts, waistlines and overall wellbeing. Some varieties can actually exacerbate many of those aggravating menopause symptoms we're so desperate to escape, like stubborn belly fat, high cholesterol, inflammation, and fatigue.

And during a life stage when our risks for developing chronic illnesses like heart disease, osteoporosis and diabetes are already heightened, we need to be extra diligent about cutting back on the fats that can potentially worsen those conditions. A little knowledge goes a long way in making smart choices.

So let's take a closer look at the two main types of unhealthy fats that are important to minimize - saturated fats and trans fats. By being more aware of where they're lurking and how they can undermine our efforts, it becomes easier to steer clear and stay on that path towards improved menopause health.

The Saturated Fat Situation

I'll admit, saturated fats and I go way back...like all the way back to my childhood. Frying bacon for my father's breakfast was one of my first cooking jobs as a kid, leaving the kitchen coated in a glistening layer of grease. Grandma's signature treats were always loaded with butter too - from her famous chocolate chip cookies to that devilishly rich cheesecake.

For decades, saturated fats held a starring role in many of our favorite comfort foods and indulgences. And while they can certainly be enjoyed in moderate amounts, boosting our intake too high can spell serious trouble during the already tricky menopause years.

You see, saturated fats are aptly named because they're solid at room temperature. Their molecular structures are saturated with hydrogen atoms, making them very resistant to going rancid. This super stability comes at a cost though - saturated fats can raise our levels of harmful LDL cholesterol more than any other fatty variety.

Research shows saturated fat also has a pro-inflammatory effect, creating metabolic conditions that increase disease risk. Not exactly what we need as estrogen depletes and our bodies grow more susceptible to issues like insulin resistance, bone loss, and cognitive decline.

To make matters worse, saturated fat has been linked to impaired sleep quality and more difficulty losing weight, two of the biggest insults we face during menopause. One study found that when people reduced saturated fat intake, they fell asleep faster and experienced deeper, more restorative slumber.

You should know that while saturated fat isn't necessarily off-limits, it calls for some major moderation. That means scaling way back on fatty cuts of meat, heavily marbled steaks, poultry with the skin left on, whole milk dairy products, butter, cheese, and anything fried in partially hydrogenated vegetable oil.

Many baked goods and processed snacks like chips, crackers, and frozen meals are shockingly high in saturated fat as well. So be diligent about checking nutrition labels and opting for healthier whole food fats instead, like those from avocados, nuts and olive oil.

The Truth About Trans Fats

But if there's one variety of fat we absolutely want to cut out of our menopausal diets as much as humanly possible, it would have to be artificial trans fats. These franken fats are considered the worst of the worst - a total monster when it comes to increasing our risks for heart disease, stroke, inflammation and weight gain.

Trans fats are born through an insidious process called hydrogenation, in which hydrogen molecules are artificially added to liquid vegetable oils to make them solid at room temp and resistant to spoiling. This alteration extends shelf life while creating that waxy, creamy texture we all know from hydrogenated shortenings, stick margarine and certain fried foods.

But here's the catch - our bodies cannot metabolize these chemically-altered fats properly, wreaking total havoc on our cells in the process. Trans fats not only increase LDL cholesterol levels while decreasing the beneficial HDLs, they create systemic inflammation that can trigger or worsen a myriad of diseases and conditions.

In fact, trans fats from partially hydrogenated oils are so physiologically damaging that the FDA has actually ruled them to be unsafe for consumption. Food manufacturers have until 2023 to eliminate them from products completely, though many have already started phasing them out in response to increased consumer awareness about their dangers.

For any woman dealing with the hormonal upheaval of menopause, consuming trans fats only exacerbates things further. Their impact on inflammatory processes and cholesterol levels can spell big trouble for our heart, bones, and brains at a time when those tissues are already more vulnerable. Not to mention that trans fats make it incredibly difficult to maintain a healthy weight by interfering with our bodies' natural satiety signals.

So where might these sneaky, shape-shifting fats still be lurking? The usual culprits include many fried items like French fries and doughnuts, certain pie crusts and biscuits, frozen foods like pizzas and microwave dinners, refrigerator doughs, chips and crackers, and cookies, cakes and other baked goods containing partially hydrogenated oils. Basically, any product that contains the words "hydrogenated oil" or "partially hydrogenated oil" is fair game for those metabolic terrorists.

Fortunately, as consumers have grown more educated and started avoiding them in droves, trans fat levels in the food supply have dropped considerably. But they're still not completely extinct yet, which means we've got to remain diligent about checking nutrition labels and steering clear.

The Balancing Act

Now, none of this is to say that every last saturated or trans-fat has to be expunged from our lives entirely. I could never realistically quit cheese or peanut butter altogether, and I wouldn't want to live in a world without the occasional French fry indulgence!

What's key is maintaining an overall balanced diet that emphasizes good unsaturated sources like olive oil, avocados, nuts and seafood while enjoying those more menopause-unfriendly varieties in strict moderation. For example, the saturated fat in a small amount of butter to cook with or drizzle of heavy cream in a sauce would be no big deal.

But downing fast food milkshakes, mainlining potato chips, and pan-frying our proteins in heaps of oil day after day after day? Now that's a straight shot towards weight gain, chronic inflammation, hormone disruption and many of those other symptoms we're all so desperate to escape. A little mindfulness can help.

By keeping unhealthy saturated and trans fats to a bare minimum while loading up on those good monounsaturated, polyunsaturated and omega-3 fatty acid sources, we're giving our bodies an incredible advantage during this transitional phase. Our hormones, hearts, bones, and metabolisms will stay more resilient and robust as we move through menopause changes with grace.

let's embrace fat in all of its nourishing, health-promoting forms while saying "see ya" to the sneaky saboteurs. Our plates are about to get a whole lot more delicious while keeping us feeling cool, calm and balanced in the process! Next up, we'll cover the very best quality fat sources to stock your kitchen with.

Chapter 2: Fats for Menopause Symptom Relief

I will never forget the first time I experienced a full-blown menopausal hot flash. One minute, I was totally fine, prepping ingredients for our family taco night like any other evening. The next, sweat started pouring down my face and back like I was a gallon jug of water someone had knocked over. My clothes became drenched and stuck to my skin as an intense wave of body heat just radiated outwards.

Of course, this wasn't an isolated occurrence. Those prickly sensations of smoldering from the inside out quickly became the banes of my existence, frequently sabotaging even the most mundane daily activities. Hot flashes could strike at any given moment without warning - during a work meeting, while running errands, even in the depths of the night leaving me shaking from the chills afterwards.

There I'd be, trying in vain to discretely fan myself and crank up the AC, praying that my flaming red face wouldn't betray my discomfort to whoever was around me. Yet beneath those visible hot flash pyrotechnics, a deeper level of hormonal havoc was brewing, leaving me increasingly moody, foggy-brained, and perpetually depleted on the energy front too.

But amid all that misery, I finally caught a lifeline in the form of some very nourishing little fats and oils - those same healthy varieties we discussed in the previous chapter. By purposefully boosting my intake of omega-3s, monounsaturated fats, and other plant-based oils, I was able to gain some semblance of control back over my most persistent menopause woes.

How Healthy Fats Reduce Hot Flashes & Night Sweats

If you've ever witnessed someone in the throes of a menopausal hot flash, those fiery sensations can certainly seem extreme from an outsider's perspective. But they actually start from a very internal place - our hormones and the intricate chemical balancing act happening in our brains and bodies.

You see, estrogen plays a pivotal role in regulating our body temperatures at a molecular level, acting as a powerful coolant of sorts. But as our estrogen supplies become erratic and depleted during menopause, those internal thermostats directing our heat distribution go haywire too.

In the absence of estrogen's stabilizing effects, certain brain chemicals like norepinephrine and serotonin can trigger exaggerated heat production and severe hot flashes seemingly out of the blue. Those elevated temperatures then bring on night sweats and insomnia too.

The good news is that healthy fats rich in omega-3 fatty acids act like hormone regulators, producing cooling, calming effects throughout our systems. They help modulate estrogen production while influencing those neurotransmitters like serotonin implicated in hot flashes. Simply put, omega-3s assist in restoring normal temperature control. Numerous clinical trials have demonstrated omega-3s' hot flash-reducing capabilities. Women who increased their omega-3 consumption from foods like fatty fish, walnuts, and flaxseeds reported experiencing both fewer and less intense hot flashes than those not incorporating these fats regularly. Some studies saw reductions in night sweat frequency as high as 50%.

Healthy fats can't completely eliminate hot flashes or other hormonal symptoms, but they provide remarkable natural relief. Plus, their benefits extend beyond promoting better temperature regulation too.

Fats for Fighting Mood Swings & Brain Fog

For me, some of the most challenging and unexpected aspects of menopause started happening upstairs, mentally speaking. What I once chalked up to merely having a "blonde moment" or "mommy brain" quickly escalated to bouts of disconcerting forgetfulness, mental fatigue, anxiety and unpredictable mood swings.

One minute I'd be totally fine, then a dark cloud would roll in, leaving me feeling irritable and irrationally angry over the smallest things. Some days, important thoughts and words would simply evaporate from my mind mid-sentence, hampering my ability to communicate properly. Staying focused on tasks felt next to impossible as that nagging brain fog descended.

If this all sounds dreadfully familiar, you can take heart in knowing that good fats offer valuable support here too. For starters, their dense payloads of omega-3s have been proven to elevate mood and reduce depression, anxiety, and mood disorder risk during the menopausal transition.

That's because our brains are primarily comprised of fat, requiring a steady supply of those essential fatty acids to maintain stable hormone levels and prevent inflammation from mucking things up. Omega-3 DHA in particular is a major building block for brain cell membranes and healthy neurotransmitter activity.

Meanwhile, monounsaturated fats' ability to modulate blood sugar and keep energy levels stable can significantly improve focus, concentration, and memory. Fat sources like avocados, olive oil, and nut butters help optimize our glucose metabolism to keep brains firing on all cylinders rather than sputtering.

So, loading up on these cognition-protecting healthy fats may help clear out that foggy haze and rebalance those erratic mood swings from a nutritional basis. But wait, there are still more symptom-soothing benefits to cover!

Fats to Fight Fatigue

Of all the menopausal side effects I've dealt with, the constant barrage of fatigue and listlessness has been particularly draining, no pun intended. It's like no amount of sleep is ever restorative and simply getting through each day requires enormous mental effort.

Yet within a couple weeks of purposefully increasing my intake of healthy fats, I felt that heavy veil of tiredness start to lift. It was as though my body had finally received the proper nourishment for hormonal balance and my energy stores were replenishing themselves.

In fact, loads of scientific research touts omega-3s, monounsaturated fats, and other plant-based oils for their natural energizing effects during menopause. Their secret lies in promoting more efficient mitochondrial function at the cellular level - these are our cells' energy powerhouses where all metabolic activities are carried out.

Giving our mitochondria premium fuel sources like omega-3s essentially turbo-charges our entire energy production cycle. By helping our cells extract more usable energy from the foods we eat, less goes to waste. Antioxidant compounds in healthy oils are also believed to exert fatigue-fighting effects.

Additionally, menopause tends to trigger physiological changes that zap our stamina and productivity. Estrogen decline makes us more prone to inflammation, sleep disturbances, and insulin resistance, all of which feed into that overwhelming feeling of lethargy.

But high-quality fats can give us a leg up on battling those energy vampires too. Their omega fatty acids tamp down inflammation, while monounsaturated fats improve insulin sensitivity for stable blood sugar regulation. Quality sleep naturally follows to further bolster our pep.

So what are some of the tastiest energy-promoting fat sources to keep on hand? Salmon and other fatty fish deliver those coveted omega-3s EPA and DHA crucial for hormone balance and antioxidant activities. Walnuts, chia and flax seeds offer ALA, the plant-derived omega-3 that converts to EPA and DHA.

Then you've got your monounsaturated fat heavy-hitters like avocados, olive oil, almonds and almond butter, cashews and cashew butter, pecans, pistachios, peanuts and peanut butter - all absolutely loaded with fatigue-fighting powers. And don't forget about the polyunsaturated plant oils like walnut, sesame, grapeseed, and pumpkin seed oils either.

By combining a variety of these healthy fat sources into your daily routine, you'll be giving your menopausal body an incredible energy boost from the inside out. Those sluggish, irritable, and foggy experiences will gradually be replaced by vibrance and clarity as hormones stabilize and mitochondria start firing on all cylinders again.

So let's sideline the struggles over hot flashes, mood issues, and fatigue. With the wisdom of good fats on our side, we can start managing our most aggravating symptoms from the very meals we're eating. It's a delicious start towards reclaiming our vitality!

Next up, we'll cover how healthy dietary fats can be our biggest weight loss allies during menopause and provide tips for incorporating them into meals. But for now, I'd love to hear how fats are already making an impact on your menopause experience so far. The struggle is real...but so is the solution!

Recipes

Avocado Smoothie

Prep Time: 5 minutes
Cook Time: 0 minutes
Servings: 1

Ingredients:
- 1 ripe avocado, pitted and flesh scooped out
- 1 cup unsweetened almond milk
- 1 banana
- 2 tbsp old-fashioned oats
- 1 tbsp ground flaxseed
- 1 tsp honey (optional)

Directions:
1. Add all ingredients to a blender and blend until completely smooth and creamy.
2. Pour into a glass and enjoy immediately.

Nutrition:
Calories: 470, Fat: 32g (8g saturated), Protein: 9g, Carbs: 44g, Fiber: 14g

Dietary Notes: Vegan, Gluten-Free, Dairy-Free

Salmon Veggie Packets

**Prep Time: 10 minutes Cook Time: 20 minutes
Servings: 4**

Ingredients:
- 4 (6 oz) salmon fillets
- 2 cups broccoli florets
- 1 cup sliced bell peppers
- 1 cup sliced zucchini
- 2 tbsp olive oil
- 2 tsp lemon juice
- 2 cloves garlic, minced
- Salt and pepper to taste

Directions:
1. Preheat oven to 400°F.
2. Make 4 foil packet squares.
3. In each packet, layer 1/4 of the veggies. Top with a salmon fillet.
4. Drizzle each packet with 1/2 tbsp olive oil, 1/2 tsp lemon juice, garlic, salt and pepper.
5. Seal packets and place on a baking sheet.
6. Bake for 18-20 minutes until salmon is cooked through.

Nutrition (per packet):
Calories: 340, Fat: 20g (3.5g saturated), Protein: 34g, Carbs: 10g, Fiber: 4g

Dietary Notes: Gluten-Free, Dairy-Free

Coconut Vegetable Curry

**Prep Time: 15 minutes Cook Time: 30 minutes
Servings: 4**

Ingredients:

- 1 tbsp coconut oil
- 1 onion, diced
- 3 cloves garlic, minced
- 1 tbsp grated ginger
- 2 tbsp red curry paste
- 1 (13.5 oz) can coconut milk
- 1 cup vegetable or chicken broth
- 1 red bell pepper, sliced
- 2 cups cauliflower florets
- 1 cup green beans, trimmed
- 1/4 cup cashews
- 2 tbsp lime juice
- Salt to taste
- Chopped cilantro for garnish

Directions:

1. In a large pot, heat the coconut oil over medium heat.
2. Add the onion and cook 2-3 minutes until translucent.
3. Add the garlic, ginger, and curry paste. Cook 1 minute until fragrant.
4. Pour in the coconut milk and broth. Add the bell pepper, cauliflower, and green beans.
5. Bring to a boil, then reduce heat and simmer 15-20 minutes until veggies are tender.
6. Remove from heat and stir in cashews and lime juice. Season with salt.
7. Serve over rice or cauliflower rice. Garnish with cilantro.

Nutrition (1/4 of recipe):

Calories: 360, Fat: 29g (17g saturated), Protein: 8g, Carbs: 22g, Fiber: 6g

Notes: Vegan, Gluten-Free, Dairy-Free

Walnut Pesto Zucchini Noodles

**Prep Time: 15 minutes Cook Time: 0 minutes
Servings: 2**

Ingredients:
- 2 medium zucchinis, spiralized into noodles
- 1 cup fresh basil leaves
- 1/2 cup toasted walnuts
- 1/4 cup olive oil
- 2 cloves garlic
- 2 tbsp lemon juice
- 1/4 cup grated parmesan cheese (omit for vegan)
- Salt and pepper to taste

Directions:
1. Make the pesto by blending the basil, walnuts, olive oil, garlic, lemon juice, and parmesan (if using) in a food processor until smooth. Season with salt and pepper.
2. Toss the zucchini noodles with the desired amount of pesto until fully coated.
3. Allow to marinate for 5-10 minutes before serving.
4. Top with extra walnuts if desired.

Nutrition (1/2 of recipe):
Calories: 560, Fat: 52g (7g saturated), Protein: 12g, Carbs: 16g, Fiber: 5g

Notes: Vegetarian, Gluten-Free. Omit parmesan for Vegan

Nutty Overnight Oats

**Prep Time: 5 minutes (plus overnight) Cook Time:
0 minutes
Servings: 1**

Ingredients:
- 1/2 cup old-fashioned oats
- 1/2 cup unsweetened almond milk
- 1/4 cup plain Greek yogurt
- 1 tbsp ground flaxseed
- 1 tbsp nut butter (almond, peanut, etc.)
- 1 tsp honey or maple syrup
- 1/4 tsp vanilla extract
- 1/4 cup fresh or frozen berries

Directions:
1. In a jar or bowl, combine the oats, almond milk, yogurt, flaxseed, nut butter, sweetener, and vanilla.
2. Mix well until fully combined.
3. Cover and refrigerate overnight.
4. In the morning, remove from fridge and top with berries.

Nutrition:
Calories: 390, Fat: 18g (2g saturated), Protein: 17g, Carbs: 46g, Fiber: 10g

Notes: Vegetarian, Gluten-Free

Chapter 3: Fats for Weight Management

I think we can all agree that one of the most frustrating side effects of menopause is the dreadful battle of the bulge. No matter how diligently I watched my calorie intake or spent hours sweating it out at the gym, the pounds just seemed to accumulate in all the wrong places. My once trim waistline was thickening up, my clothes felt skin-tight, and the number on the scale kept infuriatingly rising.

If this sounds anything like your experience, please know you're definitely not alone. Up to 90% of women struggle with menopause weight gain, no matter their usual body type or activity levels beforehand. All those hormonal fluctuations hitting our metabolisms make losing weight incredibly difficult during this transition.

Yet stepping on the scale isn't just about pursuing an idealized body shape or size. Excess weight, especially around the abdomen, significantly increases our risks for a slew of serious health issues like heart disease, stroke, type 2 diabetes, and even certain cancers too. Not great odds when our chances of developing those chronic conditions are already heightened postmenopausally.

So clearly, managing our menopause weight is about far more than just looking good in a swimsuit. It's absolutely crucial for protecting our long-term wellbeing too. But no one ever said it would be easy! Fortunately, doubling down on healthy fats can give us a major leg up in this uphill battle.

The Role of Healthy Fats for Feeling Full

Have you ever noticed how unsatisfying a low-fat meal can be? You polish off every bite, only to be ravenously hungry again just an hour or two later. Before you know it, you're mindlessly reaching for whatever snacks are nearby or second-helping it because you simply don't feel satiated.

That's because dietary fats are absolute rockstars when it comes to promoting a feeling of lasting fullness and crushing cravings. They stimulate satiety hormones like leptin and cholecystokinin, which signal to our brains that we've had enough to eat. Fats also slow down the digestive process so fewer blood sugar spikes and dips occur after our meals.

In contrast, highly processed foods devoid of healthy fats are metabolized rapidly, causing our blood sugar levels to spike then plummet soon after. This triggers hunger pangs, brain fog, irritability, and we go reaching for another snack in an endless cycle. Not great when we're already battling menopausal munchies from hormonal shifts.

But by making sure each meal and snack contains quality fats from avocado, olive oil, nuts, seeds and the like, we're able to sidestep those hangry episodes and unhealthy cravings. We simply feel fuller for longer and are far less likely to overeat later as a result.

Healthy fats also offer superior satiety compared to plain protein or carb sources alone. They give meals a richer, creamier consistency that satisfies our cravings for comfort foods in a way that's both nutritious and flat belly-friendly.

Case in point: baked potato topped with Greek yogurt and fresh salsa versus loaded with butter, cheese and bacon. Even though the toppings provide comparable calories, the healthy fats leave us feeling fuller for longer.

Thus, we naturally consume fewer calories overall by the end of the day.

Nutrients in Fats that Support Lean Muscle

But it's not just about feeling full and reducing overall calorie consumption. Healthy fats also play pivotal roles in preserving metabolism-revving lean muscle tissue, which tends to diminish as we get older - especially during menopause. The more muscle we can hang onto, the more calories we'll burn even at rest.

It all stems back to those changing hormones again. Lower estrogen production coupled with other physiological menopause shifts actually impairs our bodies' ability to efficiently build and maintain muscle tissue. That's not great news for our metabolic rates or strength levels.

However, getting sufficient amounts of healthy fats in our diets can help counteract this trend. That's because certain fatty acids are absolutely essential for initiating muscle protein synthesis and preventing existing muscle from breaking down.

For example, monounsaturated fatty acids (MUFAs) like those found in olive oil, avocados, and nuts directly influence pathways that preserve and build lean body mass. MUFAs enhance the muscle cell's ability to take up amino acids, while also stimulating testosterone production necessary for muscle growth and strength.

These MUFAs are also highly anti-inflammatory, warding off excessive breakdown of existing muscle tissue over time. Their abundant antioxidants are protective too, fighting cellular aging and damage that would otherwise eat away at our hard-earned muscle.

Then we've got the revered omega-3 fatty acids from fatty fish, walnuts, flax, and chia seeds.

These polyunsaturated fats are indispensable not only for heart and brain health, but for facilitating muscle recovery after exercise. They help reduce post-workout muscle soreness and inflammation.

Plus, omega-3s enhance our bodies' abilities to shuttle amino acids directly into muscle cells as they repair microscopic exercise-induced tears. Taking fish oil supplements has even been shown to increase lean muscle gains from strength training programs over a placebo.

Now I realize not all of us are vigorously hitting the weights, but many health experts recommend menopausal women do incorporate some form of regular resistance training to counteract age-related muscle loss. Whether that means lifting actual weights, doing bodyweight exercises, or working with resistance bands, every little bit of stimulus helps.

To best support these precious muscle-preserving and building efforts, we want to make sure we're generously providing our bodies with those key fats before and after our workouts. Having ample MUFAs and omega-3s available allows our muscle cells to actually utilize that exercise input to its maximum potential for growth and recovery.

So, while menopause may be continually working against us, doubling down on those growth-promoting, anti-inflammatory, recovery-enhancing fats can help swing the pendulum back in our favor. We're not only able to control our weight more easily, but do so while preserving metabolically-active lean mass too.

Simple Strategies for Incorporating More Healthy Fats
"Ok, ok, I'm convinced!" you may be thinking. "Where do I sign up for this magical muscle-preserving, metabolism-boosting, appetite-suppressing fat stuff?!"

The great news is, prioritizing healthy fats is so straightforward and perfectly aligns with many of those coveted menopausal symptom-relieving benefits we covered in the previous chapter too. It's an absolute win-win for managing weight and overall wellness.

Some of my favorite simple swaps and additions include:

- Cooking with olive oil or avocado oil instead of butter or margarine
- Using mashed avocado as a spread instead of mayo
- Snacking on a small handful of mixed nuts and seeds
- Adding nut butters, chia, ground flax, or hemp seeds to smoothies, oatmeal, or yogurt
- Enjoying salmon, sardines, or mackerel a couple times per week
- Drizzling salads and veggies with olive oil and balsamic vinegar
- Trying new recipes featuring MUFAs and omega-3s front and center

It's not about drowning everything in these fats, but making a conscious effort to incorporate sources into your routine - even in modest amounts - can make a big difference. And don't forget, healthy fats allow you to feel satisfied while naturally curbing your overall calorie intake too.

You should know that time a craving for something creamy and rich strikes, grab yourself a handful of nuts or cook up a flavorful salmon dish. Your hunger pangs and waistline will be thanking you. And your metabolism will reward you with a nice little boost as those muscle-building processes fire up!

Recipes

Eggs with Avocado Boats

**Prep Time: 10 minutes Cook Time: 10 minutes
Servings: 2**

Ingredients:
- 2 ripe avocados
- 4 eggs
- 2 tsp olive oil
- 1/4 cup crumbled feta cheese
- 2 tbsp diced tomatoes
- 1 tbsp sliced green onions
- Salt and pepper to taste

Directions:
1. Preheat oven to 400°F.
2. Cut the avocados in half lengthwise and remove the pits, leaving a hole in the center of each half.
3. Scoop out a little bit of the avocado flesh to create a larger well.
4. Place the avocado halves in a baking dish and brush the insides with olive oil. Crack 1 egg into each avocado half.
5. Bake for 15-20 minutes until the eggs are set.
6. Remove from oven and top with crumbled feta, diced tomatoes, green onions, salt and pepper.

Nutrition (per serving of 2 avocado halves):
Calories: 420, Fat: 35g (8g saturated), Protein: 16g, Carbs: 15g, Fiber: 10g

Notes: Gluten-Free, Vegetarian

Nut & Seed Trail Mix

**Prep Time: 5 minutes Cook Time: 0 minutes
Servings: 8 (1/4 cup servings)**

Ingredients:
- 1 cup raw almonds
- 1 cup raw cashews
- 1/2 cup pumpkin seeds
- 1/2 cup sunflower seeds
- 1/4 cup unsweetened shredded coconut
- 2 tbsp chia seeds
- 1 tbsp coconut oil, melted
- 1 tsp cinnamon
- 1/4 tsp salt

Directions:
1. In a large bowl, mix together the almonds, cashews, pumpkin seeds, sunflower seeds, shredded coconut and chia seeds.
2. Drizzle with the melted coconut oil and sprinkle with the cinnamon and salt. Toss to combine.
3. Store in an airtight container for up to 2 weeks.

Nutrition (per 1/4 cup serving):
Calories: 245, Fat: 21g (4g saturated), Protein: 8g, Carbs: 10g, Fiber: 4g

Notes: Vegan, Gluten-Free, Dairy-Free

Zesty Shrimp Fajitas

**Prep Time: 15 minutes Cook Time: 15 minutes
Servings: 4**

Ingredients:

- 1 lb large shrimp, peeled and deveined
- 2 tbsp olive oil, divided
- 1 red bell pepper, sliced
- 1 green bell pepper, sliced
- 1 yellow onion, sliced
- 2 cloves garlic, minced
- 1 tsp chili powder
- 1 tsp cumin
- 1/2 tsp paprika
- 1 lime, juiced
- Salt and pepper to taste
- 4 sprouted grain tortillas or lettuce wraps
- Avocado slices, for serving

Directions:

1. In a large skillet over medium-high heat, add 1 tbsp olive oil. Add the shrimp and season with salt, pepper, chili powder, cumin and paprika. Cook for 2-3 minutes per side until opaque. Remove shrimp to a plate.
2. In the same skillet, add the remaining 1 tbsp olive oil. Add the sliced peppers and onions and cook for 5-7 minutes until softened.
3. Add the garlic and cooked shrimp back to the skillet. Squeeze the juice of 1 lime over everything.
4. Serve the shrimp and veggie fajita mixture in tortillas or lettuce wraps with avocado slices on the side.

Nutrition (per serving, doesn't include tortilla):
Calories: 250, Fat: 11g (1.5g saturated), Protein: 26g, Carbs: 13g, Fiber: 4g

Notes: Gluten-Free, Dairy-Free

Salmon Avocado Rice Bowls

**Prep Time: 10 minutes Cook Time: 15 minutes
Servings: 4**

Ingredients:
- 4 (6oz) salmon fillets
- 2 cups cooked brown rice
- 2 avocados, diced
- 1 cucumber, diced
- 1 mango, diced
- 2 tbsp olive oil
- 2 tbsp rice vinegar
- 1 tsp sesame oil
- Salt and pepper to taste

Directions:
1. Preheat oven to 400°F. Place salmon fillets on a baking sheet and season with salt, pepper and 1 tbsp of the olive oil.
2. Roast for 12-15 minutes until fish is cooked through.
3. In a small bowl, whisk together the remaining 1 tbsp olive oil, rice vinegar and sesame oil for the dressing.
4. Divide the cooked brown rice between 4 bowls. Top each with a salmon fillet, avocado, cucumber and mango.
5. Drizzle the dressing over the top of each bowl.

Nutrition (per serving):
Calories: 535, Fat: 30g (5g saturated), Protein: 33g, Carbs: 37g, Fiber: 9g

Notes: Gluten-Free, Dairy-Free

Walnut Crusted Chicken Salad

**Prep Time: 15 minutes Cook Time: 15 minutes
Servings: 4**

Ingredients:
- 1 lb. boneless, skinless chicken breasts
- 1 cup walnuts, finely chopped
- 1 egg, beaten
- 2 tbsp olive oil
- 8 cups mixed greens
- 1 apple, thinly sliced
- 1/4 cup dried cranberries
- 1/4 cup crumbled feta or goat cheese
- 2 tbsp balsamic vinegar
- 1 tbsp olive oil
- Salt and pepper to taste

Directions:

1. Pound the chicken breasts to 1/2-inch thickness and season with salt and pepper.

2. Place the chopped walnuts in a shallow bowl. Dip the chicken in the beaten egg, then in the walnuts to coat both sides.

3. In a skillet over medium-high heat, warm 2 tbsp olive oil. Cook the walnut-crusted chicken for 4-5 minutes per side until cooked through.

4. Make the vinaigrette by whisking together the 1 tbsp olive oil and balsamic vinegar. Season with salt and pepper.

5. In a large bowl, toss together the greens, apple slices, dried cranberries and cheese.

6. Slice the chicken and place on top of the salad. Drizzle the vinaigrette over everything.

Nutrition (per serving):
Calories: 435, Fat: 28g (4g saturated), Protein: 30g, Carbs:
18g, Fiber: 5g

Notes: Gluten-Free

Chapter 4: Fats for Heart Health

As I sat across from my doctor going over the results of my latest physical, her expression turned quite serious. "Sharon, your cholesterol levels are elevated and your blood pressure is higher than we'd like," she said firmly. "At this stage of menopause, you're at increased risk for heart disease if we don't get things under control."

Her words felt like a punch to the gut. Sure, I knew menopause could open the door to various health issues like osteoporosis and metabolic problems. But heart disease? The frightening image of having a heart attack or stroke flooded my mind with dread.

Unfortunately, my experience is far too common these days. Declining estrogen levels during the menopause transition can dramatically alter a woman's cardiovascular risk factors in ways that endanger our heart health for years to come if left unchecked. But with some straightforward dietary adjustments, we can fight back against those menopause-related threats.

As you'll discover, strategically incorporating more of the right healthy fats into our routines ranks among the most powerful nutritional safeguards for protecting our tickers. From optimizing cholesterol profiles to controlling blood pressure, these nourishing fats offer potent cardio benefits perfectly suited for this stage of life.

Connection Between Menopause and

Increased Heart Disease Risk

Prior to reaching our late 40s and 50s, most women enjoy a degree of natural protection against heart disease due to the cardiovascular advantages provided by higher estrogen levels. This bone-preserving hormone also helps regulate cholesterol, keeping it in a healthier range.

But once we hit menopause and estrogen production plummets, that protective cloak is lifted. Suddenly, cardiovascular risk factors like cholesterol, triglyceride, and C-reactive protein (a measure of inflammation) levels have the potential for unhealthy spikes. Blood pressure is also prone to elevations, increasing our likelihood for heart attacks, strokes, and related events.

On top of that, menopause weight gain caused by hormone fluctuations and a slowing metabolism tends to further amplify heart disease risk. Excess pounds carried around the abdomen are closely linked to insulin resistance, high triglycerides, low HDL (good) cholesterol, and hypertension.

In the years immediately following menopause, statistics show a woman's risk of cardiovascular disease increases by a staggering 50%. And with heart disease consistently ranking as the 1 killer of American women, getting ahead of it during this life stage is absolutely critical for long-term vitality.

Fortunately, a diet rich in healthy fats acts as a powerful counterforce to menopause's cardiovascular impacts. It can help prevent and even reverse many of those risk factors while providing additional protective benefits.

Healthy Fat Sources That Improve Cholesterol

& Blood Pressure

When it comes to nurturing heart health during and after menopause, polyunsaturated fats and monounsaturated fats should become our new best friends. These "good" fats not only help optimize cholesterol profiles, but can meaningfully reduce blood pressure too.

Let's start with polyunsaturated omega-3 fatty acids from oily fish like salmon, mackerel, herring, sardines, and trout. These marine creatures supply two crucial forms - EPA and DHA - that demonstrate exceptional cholesterol-regulating and anti-inflammatory abilities.

Numerous studies confirm omega-3 supplements and omega-3 rich diets can significantly raise levels of heart-protective HDL cholesterol while slashing triglycerides and dangerous LDL particles. The anti-inflammatory properties of EPA and DHA help stabilize artery linings and slow plaque accumulation.

Plant sources like walnuts, flaxseeds, and chia deliver an omega-3 precursor called ALA that converts to active EPA and DHA forms. While not as potent, ALA still yields cholesterol benefits and shouldn't be overlooked.

Meanwhile, monounsaturated fats from olive oil, avocados, most nuts and nut butters act as multi-tasking cardiovascular heroes. Like omega-3s, they favorably alter cholesterol ratios by reducing LDL and increasing HDL levels. But monounsaturated fats take it a step further by actively lowering blood pressure.

The oleic acid in these plant-based oils has been shown to enhance blood vessel function and flexibility, allowing better circulation and less strain on the heart. Adding just a few servings of monounsaturated fat sources to one's diet each week can translate to meaningful reductions in diastolic and systolic readings.

Other smart fat additions for nurturing blood pressure health include sesame oil, pumpkin seeds, hemp seeds, and tahini. These provide magnesium, potassium, calcium, and other minerals known to promote vasodilation for enhanced blood flow.

therefore, whether you're looking to stave off heart disease risk factors before they start or regain control of cholesterol and hypertension already going awry, prioritizing these healthy fats sets the perfect dietary foundation. Next up, we'll cover just how seamlessly they can be incorporated into absolutely delectable heart-smart meals your entire family will love!

Sample Healthy Fat-Packed Recipes

1. Mediterranean Quinoa Salad with Salmon

**Prep Time: 20 minutes Cooking Time: 15 minutes
Serving Size: 4 servings**

Ingredients:

- 1 cup quinoa
- 2 cups water
- 1 lb. salmon fillet
- 1 cucumber, diced
- 1 bell pepper, diced
- 1/2 red onion, finely chopped
- 1/2 cup kalamata olives, halved
-
- 1/4 cup feta cheese, crumbled
- 1/4 cup fresh parsley, chopped
- 2 tablespoons olive oil
- Juice of 1 lemon
- Salt and pepper to taste

Directions:

1. Rinse quinoa under cold water. In a saucepan, bring water to a boil, add quinoa, reduce heat to low, cover, and simmer for 15 minutes. Let it sit covered for 5 minutes, then fluff with a fork.

2. Season the salmon with salt and pepper. Grill over medium heat for 5-7 minutes per side or until fully cooked. Flake into large pieces.

3. In a large bowl, combine cooked quinoa, cucumber, bell pepper, onion, olives, and parsley. Add the flaked salmon, drizzle with olive oil and lemon juice, and toss gently. Sprinkle with feta cheese.

Nutritional Value (per serving): Approximately 400 calories, 22g protein, 20g fat, 30g carbohydrates.

Food Class: Gluten-Free

2. Garlicky Avocado Toast

Prep Time: 10 minutes Cooking Time: 0 minutes
Serving Size: 2 servings

Ingredients:

- 1 large ripe avocado
- 2 cloves garlic, minced
- 2 slices whole grain bread
- 1 tablespoon olive oil
- Salt and pepper to taste
- Red pepper flakes (optional)

Directions:

1. Peel and mash the avocado in a small bowl. Mix in minced garlic, olive oil, salt, and pepper.

2. Toast the bread slices to your liking. Spread the avocado mixture evenly on each slice. Sprinkle with red pepper flakes if desired.

Nutritional Value (per serving): Approximately 300 calories, 5g protein, 20g fat, 27g carbohydrates.

Food Class: Vegan

3. Coconut Walnut Shrimp

**Prep Time: 15 minutes Cooking Time: 10 minutes
Serving Size: 4 servings**

Ingredients:

- 1 lb. large shrimp, peeled and deveined
- 1/2 cup shredded coconut
- 1/2 cup crushed walnuts
- 2 eggs, beaten
- 1 cup flour
- Salt and pepper to taste
- Oil for frying

Directions:

1. Season shrimp with salt and pepper. Dredge in flour, dip in beaten eggs, and coat with a mixture of shredded coconut and crushed walnuts.

2. Heat oil in a frying pan over medium heat. Fry shrimp until golden brown and cooked through, about 2-3 minutes per side.

Nutritional Value (per serving): Approximately 450 calories, 24g protein, 28g fat, 20g carbohydrates.

Food Class: Gluten-Free (check flour for a gluten-free alternative)

4. Mexican Black Bean & Avocado Salad

**Prep Time: 15 minutes Cooking Time: 0 minutes
Serving Size: 4 servings**

Ingredients:

- 1 can black beans, rinsed and drained
- 1 large avocado, diced
- 1 cup cherry tomatoes, halved
- 1/2 red onion, finely chopped
- 1/4 cup fresh cilantro, chopped
- Juice of 1 lime
- 2 tablespoons olive oil
- Salt and pepper to taste

Directions:

1. In a large bowl, combine black beans, avocado, cherry tomatoes, red onion, and cilantro.
2. Drizzle with lime juice and olive oil, then season with salt and pepper. Toss gently to combine.

Nutritional Value (per serving): Approximately 250 calories, 8g protein, 14g fat, 22g carbohydrates.

Food Class: Vegan, Gluten-Free

5. Pecan-Crusted Air Fryer Salmon

**Prep Time: 10 minutes Cooking Time: 10 minutes
Serving Size: 4 servings**

Ingredients:

- 4 salmon fillets (about 6 ounces each)
- 1/2 cup pecans, finely chopped
- 1 teaspoon garlic powder
- 1 teaspoon smoked paprika
- 1/2 teaspoon salt
- 1/4 teaspoon black pepper
- 1 tablespoon olive oil

Directions:

1. Preheat your air fryer to 390°F (200°C).

2. In a small bowl, mix together chopped pecans, garlic powder, smoked paprika, salt, and pepper.

3. Brush each salmon fillet with olive oil, then press the pecan mixture onto the top of each fillet to form a crust.

4. Place the salmon fillets in the air fryer basket, skin side down, and cook for 10 minutes or until the salmon is cooked through and the crust is golden.

Nutritional Value (per serving): Approximately 350 calories, 25g protein, 23g fat, 3g carbohydrates.

Food Class: Gluten-Free

6. Pumpkin Seed Pesto Zoodles

**Prep Time: 15 minutes Cooking Time: 5 minutes
Serving Size: 4 servings**

Ingredients:

- 4 medium zucchinis, spiralized into noodles
- 1/2 cup pumpkin seeds
- 1 cup fresh basil leaves
- 2 cloves garlic
- 1/2 cup grated Parmesan cheese
- 1/4 cup olive oil
- Juice of 1 lemon
- Salt and pepper to taste

Directions:

1. In a food processor, combine pumpkin seeds, basil, garlic, Parmesan, and lemon juice. Pulse until coarsely chopped.

2. While the processor is running, slowly pour in the olive oil until the mixture becomes smooth and creamy. Season with salt and pepper.

3. Place spiralized zucchini (zoodles) in a large bowl. Toss with the pumpkin seed pesto until well coated.

4. Serve immediately, or for best flavor, let the zoodles sit for about 5-10 minutes to absorb the flavors.

Nutritional Value (per serving): Approximately 290 calories, 10g protein, 23g fat, 10g carbohydrates.

Food Class: Gluten-Free, Vegetarian

Chapter 5: Fats for Brain Power

How Healthy Fats Support Cognitive Function

During Menopause

As we navigate the menopausal transition, one of the most concerning aspects is the potential impact it can have on our cognitive abilities and neurological health. Brain fog, memory lapses, difficulty concentrating, anxiety, irritability - these manifestations of hormonal changes can leave us feeling like we're losing our minds.

But rather than resigning ourselves to this fate, we can be proactive about preserving our mental clarity and emotional well-being by strategically incorporating more brain-boosting healthy fats into our diets. The right dietary fats provide widespread benefits for fortifying our grey matter against menopause-induced cognitive decline.

Our brains are comprised of a staggering 60% fat, the majority being omega-3 and omega-6 polyunsaturated fatty acids. This dense, fatty insulation wrapped around neurons facilitates efficient communication between brain cells and regulates their firing capabilities. However, as estrogen levels drop during menopause, this delicate fatty acid balance becomes disrupted.

With estrogen's protective effects diminished, the brain becomes more vulnerable to inflammation and oxidative stress that can damage neurons and synaptic pathways critical for memory formation, information processing, mood regulation and more. Dysregulated hormones also throw levels of the stress hormone cortisol into disarray, impairing concentration and exacerbating anxiety.

This is where increasing your intake of healthy fats can make a world of difference. They serve as anti-inflammatory agents, counteracting menopause-related immune responses that muddle our cognitive capabilities. Their antioxidant properties neutralize free radicals and prevent them from accumulating in memory and mood centers of the brain.

For example, monounsaturated fatty acids found in avocados, olive oil and nuts enhance neural plasticity - the brain's ability to forge new neural connections and pathways. This allows for faster processing speeds and better retention of information, counteracting memory deficits often experienced during menopause.

The omega-3 polyunsaturated fats EPA and DHA in salmon, sardines and other fatty fish are superstars for boosting overall brain health. They not only support memory and focus by facilitating rapid neurotransmission between cells, but DHA specifically aids the brain's housekeeping systems responsible for clearing out inflammatory toxins that could otherwise accumulate.

Then you have healthy fats like those in coconut oil and grass-fed dairy products containing unique medium-chain triglycerides (MCTs). These MCT fats have been shown to reduce inflammation while improving cognitive performance, concentration and brain energy levels when the body metabolizes them into ketones.

By consuming more of these cognition-supporting fatty acids and antioxidants, we're essentially supplying our brains premium-grade fuel to run optimally despite the challenges of menopause. Inflammation and oxidative stress get extinguished before disrupting normal neural function, while critical mood-regulating chemicals remain properly synthesized.

The end result is better preservation of our memory faculties, sharper focus, stabilized moods, and an overall enhanced capacity for clear, levelheaded thinking - a welcomed reprieve from menopause brain fog!

Top Fat Sources for Improving Memory, Concentration, and Mood

Now that we understand just how instrumental healthy fats are for cognitive resilience during the menopausal transition, let's look at which specific sources we should be emphasizing.

For supporting memory function and concentration, fatty fish like salmon, mackerel, sardines, anchovies and trout are nutritional superstars. These cold-water creatures are loaded with the omega-3 fatty acids EPA and DHA, which demonstrate powerful neuroprotective and anti-inflammatory effects in the brain.

Higher omega-3 blood levels are consistently associated with enhanced brain structure, cerebral blood flow, and working memory performance in aging adults. Conversely, participants with suboptimal omega-3 status show impairments in focus, information processing speed, recall and other executive functions.

 enjoying a few servings of salmon, mackerel or sardines each week can go a long way towards sharpening your cognitive prowess. But for those who don't consume fish regularly, plant sources like chia, flaxseeds and walnuts provide a form of omega-3 called ALA that still yields memory and concentration benefits.

When it comes to mood regulation and emotional balance, monounsaturated fats and specific polyunsaturated fats should be prioritized.

Avocados are an excellent example as they contain monounsaturated fatty acids shown to support serotonin and dopamine production - those "feel-good" neurotransmitters responsible for positive mindset and outlook.

Higher avocado intake has been associated with greater resilience against anxiety, stress, depression and other neurological mood disorders. The healthy fats and nutrients in avocados appear to help stabilize hormone levels and ease menopause-related irritability too.

Similarly, walnut intake and their oils have gained attention for combating brain fog, mood swings, fatigue and other cognitive effects of menopause. Walnuts rank among the best plant sources of anti-inflammatory omega-3 ALA fats. But they also provide polyphenol antioxidants that enhance neuronal signaling pathways to improve focus and mental performance.

Coconut and its oil have also been revered for their cognition-boosting effects, particularly the medium-chain triglycerides (MCTs) they contain. These unique fats produce ketones that serve as an alternative energy source for the brain, one that's been shown to suppress inflammation and oxidative stress responsible for sluggish thinking and low mood.

Lastly, let's not forget about other mood-supporting sources of healthy unsaturated fats like nuts, seeds and their nutrient-dense oils. Cashews, pecans, pepitas, sesame and sunflower seeds deliver feel-good minerals like magnesium, zinc and vitamin E that promote balanced neurotransmitter production. Their anti-inflammatory properties also protect against hormonal mood swings. The bottom line: prioritizing an array of these brain-sharpening, cognition-protecting healthy fats should be considered self-care for the mind during the menopausal transition.

Every bite packs a wealth of antioxidants, anti-inflammatory compounds and raw materials for optimizing neurological function.

While menopause may temporarily muddle our cerebral clarity, committing to a fat-rich dietary pattern allows us to reclaim our mental superpowers! No more feeling scattered, forgetful or derailed by menopause brain fog. Instead, we rewrite the narrative around healthy aging by nurturing razor-sharp cognitive stamina for the long haul.

Recipes

Blueberry Almond Smoothie

Preparation Time: 5 minutes Cooking Time: None

Serving Size: 1 serving

Ingredients:

- 1 cup fresh blueberries
- 1/2 banana
- 1/4 cup almonds
- 1 cup almond milk
- 1 tablespoon honey (optional)
- Ice cubes (optional)

Directions:

1. Combine all ingredients in a blender.

2. Blend on high until smooth.

3. Pour into a glass and serve immediately.

Nutritional Value: (per serving)

Calories: 210 Protein: 4g Fat: 9g Carbohydrates: 30g
Fiber: 5g

Food Class: Vegan, Gluten-free

Salmon Avocado Rice Bowl

Preparation Time: 10 minutes Cooking Time: 20 minutes

Serving Size: 2 servings

Ingredients:

- 2 salmon fillets (4 oz each)
- 1 cup cooked brown rice
- 1 avocado, sliced
- 1/2 cucumber, sliced
- 2 tablespoons soy sauce
- 1 teaspoon sesame oil
- 1 tablespoon sesame seeds
- Salt and pepper to taste

Directions:

1. Season salmon with salt and pepper and cook in a preheated oven at 375°F for about 15-20 minutes.

2. In two bowls, place an equal amount of rice.

3. Top rice with cooked salmon, avocado slices, and cucumber.

4. Drizzle with soy sauce and sesame oil.

5. Sprinkle sesame seeds on top and serve.

Nutritional Value: (per serving)

Calories: 650 Protein: 25g Fat: 35g Carbohydrates: 55g

Fiber: 7g

Food Class: Gluten-free

Trail Mix Energy Bites

**Preparation Time: 15 minutes Cooking Time: None
Serving Size: 12 bites**

Ingredients:

- 1 cup rolled oats
- 1/2 cup peanut butter
- 1/4 cup honey
- 1/4 cup dried cranberries
- 1/4 cup chocolate chips
- 1/4 cup chopped almonds

Directions:

1. In a bowl, mix all ingredients until well combined.

2. Roll the mixture into balls, each about the size of a walnut.

3. Refrigerate for at least an hour before serving.

Nutritional Value: (per bite)

Calories: 150 Protein: 4g Fat: 8g Carbohydrates: 18g

Fiber: 2g

Food Class: Vegetarian, Gluten-free

Chapter 6: Breakfast

Easy, Nutrient-Dense, High-Fat Breakfast

Recipes

Avocado Toast with Egg

Prep Time: 10 minutes Serving Size: 1

Ingredients:

- 1 slice whole-grain bread
- 1/2 ripe avocado, mashed
- 1 egg, cooked as desired
- Sea salt and black pepper, to taste
- Red pepper flakes (optional)

Directions:

1. Toast the bread slice.

2. Mash the avocado and spread it over the toasted bread.

3. Top with the cooked egg and season with salt, pepper, and red pepper flakes (if desired).

Nutritional Value: High in healthy fats, protein, fiber, and various vitamins and minerals.

Food Class: Can be made vegan by omitting the egg.

Chia Pudding with Mixed Berries

Prep Time: 5 minutes (plus overnight soaking)
Serving Size: 1

Ingredients:

- 1/4 cup chia seeds
- 1 cup unsweetened almond milk
- 1 tablespoon maple syrup (optional)
- 1/2 teaspoon vanilla extract
- 1 cup mixed berries

Directions:

1. In a jar or bowl, combine the chia seeds, almond milk, maple syrup (if using), and vanilla extract. Stir well.

2. Cover and refrigerate overnight (or for at least 4 hours) to allow the chia seeds to swell and form a pudding-like consistency.

3. Top with mixed berries before serving.

Nutritional Value: High in fiber, healthy fats, antioxidants, and plant-based protein.

Food Class: Vegan, gluten-free.

Smoked Salmon and Cream Cheese Stuffed

Avocado

Prep Time: 10 minutes Serving Size: 1

Ingredients:

- 1 ripe avocado
- 2 ounces smoked salmon
- 2 tablespoons cream cheese
- 1 tablespoon chopped fresh dill
- Lemon wedges for serving

Directions:

1. Cut the avocado in half lengthwise and remove the pit.

2. In a small bowl, mix together the smoked salmon, cream cheese, and dill.

3. Divide the salmon mixture evenly between the two avocado halves, stuffing it into the pits.

4. Serve with lemon wedges on the side.

Nutritional Value: High in healthy fats, protein, and various vitamins and minerals.

Food Class: Gluten-free, can be made dairy-free by using a plant-based cream cheese alternative.

Almond Butter and Banana Smoothie

Prep Time: 5 minutes Serving Size: 1

Ingredients:

- 1 ripe banana
- 2 tablespoons almond butter
- 1 cup unsweetened almond milk
- 1/2 teaspoon ground cinnamon
- 1/4 teaspoon vanilla extract (optional)

Directions:

1. Add all ingredients to a blender and blend until smooth.

2. Pour into a glass and enjoy!

Nutritional Value: High in healthy fats, fiber, protein, and various vitamins and minerals.

Food Class: Vegan, gluten-free.

Spinach and Feta Egg Muffins

**Prep Time: 15 minutes Cook Time: 20 minutes
Serving Size: 6 muffins**

Ingredients:

- 6 eggs
- 1/4 cup milk (or plant-based milk alternative)
- 1/2 cup crumbled feta cheese
- 1 cup fresh spinach, chopped
- 1/4 cup chopped sun-dried tomatoes
- Salt and pepper, to taste

Directions:

1. Preheat the oven to 350°F (175°C). Grease a 6-cup muffin tin.
2. In a bowl, whisk together the eggs and milk. Season with salt and pepper.
3. Stir in the feta cheese, spinach, and sun-dried tomatoes.
4. Evenly distribute the egg mixture into the prepared muffin cups.
5. Bake for 18-20 minutes, or until the egg muffins are set and golden brown on top.
6. Let cool for 5 minutes before serving.

Nutritional Value: High in protein, healthy fats, and various vitamins and minerals.

Food Class: Gluten-free, vegetarian.

Coconut Chia Pudding with Mango

Prep Time: 5 minutes (plus overnight soaking)
Serving Size: 1

Ingredients:

- 1/4 cup chia seeds
- 1 cup unsweetened coconut milk
- 1 tablespoon honey or maple syrup (optional)
- 1/2 teaspoon vanilla extract
- 1 ripe mango, diced

Directions:

1. In a jar or bowl, combine the chia seeds, coconut milk, honey/maple syrup (if using), and vanilla extract. Stir well.

2. Cover and refrigerate overnight (or for at least 4 hours) to allow the chia seeds to swell and form a pudding-like consistency.

3. Top with diced mango before serving.

Nutritional Value: High in fiber, healthy fats, antioxidants, and plant-based protein.

Food Class: Vegan, gluten-free.

Loaded Veggie Frittata

Prep Time: 15 minutes Cook Time: 25 minutes
Serving Size: 4

Ingredients:

- 8 eggs
- 1/4 cup milk (or plant-based milk alternative)
- 1/2 cup diced bell peppers
- 1/2 cup diced onions
- 1 cup fresh spinach, chopped
- 1/2 cup sliced mushrooms
- 1/4 cup crumbled feta cheese (optional)
- Salt and pepper, to taste

Directions:

1. Preheat the oven to 350°F (175°C). Grease an oven-safe skillet or baking dish.
2. In a bowl, whisk together the eggs and milk. Season with salt and pepper.
3. In the prepared skillet or baking dish, arrange the bell peppers, onions, spinach, and mushrooms in an even layer.
4. Pour the egg mixture over the vegetables.
5. Sprinkle the feta cheese on top (if using).
6. Bake for 20-25 minutes, or until the frittata is set and golden brown on top.
7. Let cool for 5 minutes before slicing and serving.

Nutritional Value: High in protein, fiber, and various vitamins and minerals.

Food Class: Can be made vegetarian by omitting the feta cheese, or vegan by using a plant-based milk alternative and omitting the feta cheese.

Yogurt Parfaits

Prep Time: 10 minutes Serving Size: 1

- 1 cup Greek yogurt (plain or vanilla)
- 1/2 cup mixed berries (fresh or frozen)
- 2 tablespoons granola
- 1 tablespoon sliced almonds
- 1 teaspoon honey (optional)

Directions:

1. In a parfait glass or jar, layer half of the yogurt, followed by half of the mixed berries.

2. Top with half of the granola and almonds.

3. Repeat the layers with the remaining yogurt, berries, granola, and almonds.

4. Drizzle with honey if desired.

Nutritional Value: High in protein, healthy fats, fiber, and various vitamins and minerals from the yogurt, berries, nuts, and seeds.

Food Class: Gluten-free, vegetarian (can be made vegan by using plant-based yogurt and omitting honey).

Zucchini Frittata

**Prep Time: 15 minutes Cook Time: 25 minutes
Serving Size: 4**

Ingredients:

- 8 eggs
- 1/4 cup milk (or plant-based milk alternative)
- 1 cup grated zucchini
- 1/2 cup diced bell peppers
- 1/4 cup crumbled feta cheese (optional)
- 2 tablespoons chopped fresh herbs (e.g., parsley, dill, or basil)
- Salt and pepper, to taste

Directions:

1. Preheat the oven to 350°F (175°C). Grease an oven-safe skillet or baking dish.

2. In a bowl, whisk together the eggs and milk. Season with salt and pepper.

3. Stir in the grated zucchini, bell peppers, feta cheese (if using), and fresh herbs.

4. Pour the egg mixture into the prepared skillet or baking dish.

5. Bake for 20-25 minutes, or until the frittata is set and golden brown on top.

6. Let cool for 5 minutes before slicing and serving.

Nutritional Value: High in protein, fiber, and various vitamins and minerals from the eggs, vegetables, and cheese (if used).

Chocolate Hazelnut Smoothie

Prep Time: 5 minutes Serving Size: 1

Ingredients:

- 1 ripe banana
- 1 cup unsweetened almond milk
- 2 tablespoons hazelnut butter
- 2 tablespoons cocoa powder
- 1 tablespoon honey or maple syrup (optional)
- 1/2 teaspoon vanilla extract (optional)

Directions:

1. Add all ingredients to a blender and blend until smooth and creamy.

2. Pour into a glass and enjoy!

Nutritional Value: High in healthy fats, fiber, protein, and various vitamins and minerals from the nuts, banana, and cocoa powder.

Food Class: Vegan, gluten-free.

Meal Prep Tips for Grab-and-Go Options

Meal prepping breakfast options is a great way to ensure you have nutrient-dense, high-fat options ready to grab and go on busy mornings. Here are some valuable tips for meal prepping breakfast:

1. Batch Cooking: Prepare breakfast items in batches on the weekend or at the beginning of the week. Frittatas, egg muffins, chia puddings, and overnight oats are perfect for batch cooking and portioning out for the week ahead.

2. Portable Containers: Invest in high-quality, leak-proof containers or jars to store your prepped breakfast items. Mason jars are great for parfaits, chia puddings, and overnight oats, while bento-style containers work well for frittatas, egg muffins, and avocado toast ingredients.

3. Freezer-Friendly Options: Some breakfast items, like frittatas, egg muffins, and smoothie packs (pre-portioned and frozen), can be prepared in advance and frozen for longer storage. Thaw them overnight in the refrigerator or grab them straight from the freezer and reheat or blend them in the morning.

4. Prep Ingredients Ahead: Chop and portion out ingredients like vegetables, fruits, nuts, and seeds in advance. This makes it easier to assemble grab-and-go options quickly in the morning or for the next few days.

5. Freezer-Friendly Options: Some breakfast items, like frittatas, egg muffins, and smoothie packs (pre-portioned and frozen), can be prepared in advance and frozen for longer storage. Thaw them overnight in the refrigerator or grab them straight from the freezer and reheat or blend them in the morning. Baked goods like muffins, breakfast cookies, and energy balls can also be frozen and thawed or

reheated as needed. Additionally, you can portion out ingredients for smoothies (like frozen fruit, spinach, etc.) into individual bags or containers and store them in the freezer for quick blending.

6. Rotation and Variety: To keep things interesting and prevent burnout, rotate different breakfast options throughout the week or month. You can also mix and match ingredients to create new flavor combinations.

7. Overnight Preparations: For items like overnight oats, chia puddings, and parfaits, prepare them the night before and refrigerate them, so they're ready to grab and go in the morning.

8. Batch Cook Proteins: Cook large batches of proteins like hard-boiled eggs, turkey bacon, or chicken sausage, and portion them out for easy addition to breakfast dishes or sandwiches.

9. Stay Organized: Label containers with the contents and date, and keep a running inventory of what you have prepped to avoid waste and ensure you're rotating through your stock.

10. Repurpose Leftovers: Get creative with repurposing dinner leftovers (like roasted vegetables, quinoa, or shredded meats) into breakfast dishes like frittatas, breakfast burritos, or bowls.

By incorporating these meal prep tips, you'll have a variety of nutrient-dense, high-fat breakfast options readily available, making it easier to start your day with a nourishing meal, even on the busiest of mornings.

Fresh Salad Recipes Showcasing Healthy Fats

Spinach Salad with Warm Bacon Vinaigrette

Prep Time: 15 minutes Serving Size: 4

Ingredients:

- 8 cups fresh spinach
- 4 slices bacon, diced
- 1 small shallot, minced
- 2 tablespoons red wine vinegar
- 1 tablespoon Dijon mustard
- 2 tablespoons olive oil
- 1/4 cup crumbled feta cheese (optional)
- Salt and pepper, to taste

Directions:

1. Cook the bacon in a skillet over medium heat until crispy. Remove bacon from the skillet, reserving the bacon fat.
2. Add the minced shallot to the bacon fat and sauté for 1 minute.
3. Remove from heat and whisk in the red wine vinegar, Dijon mustard, and olive oil.
4. Season with salt and pepper to taste.
5. In a large bowl, toss the spinach with the warm bacon vinaigrette and crumbled feta cheese (if using).
6. Top with the crispy bacon bits and serve immediately.

Kale and Quinoa Salad with Avocado Dressing

Prep Time: 20 minutes Serving Size: 4

Ingredients:

- 4 cups kale, chopped
- 1 cup cooked quinoa
- 1 avocado
- 2 tablespoons lemon juice
- 2 tablespoons olive oil
- 1/4 cup toasted almonds
- Salt and pepper, to taste

Directions:

1. In a large bowl, combine the chopped kale and cooked quinoa.
2. In a blender or food processor, combine the avocado, lemon juice, olive oil, and a pinch of salt and pepper. Blend until smooth and creamy.
3. Pour the avocado dressing over the kale and quinoa mixture, and toss to combine.
4. Top with toasted almonds before serving.

Nutritional Value: High in healthy fats, fiber, plant-based protein, and various vitamins and minerals.

Food Class: Vegan, gluten-free.

Grilled Peach and Burrata Salad

**Prep Time: 15 minutes Cook Time: 5 minutes
Serving Size: 4**

Ingredients:

- 4 ripe peaches, halved and pitted
- 8 ounces burrata cheese
- 4 cups mixed greens
- 1/4 cup toasted walnuts
- 2 tablespoons balsamic glaze
- 2 tablespoons olive oil
- Salt and pepper, to taste

Directions:

1. Preheat a grill or grill pan over medium-high heat.
2. Brush the cut sides of the peach halves with a little olive oil and grill for 2-3 minutes per side, until slightly charred.
3. In a large bowl, combine the mixed greens, grilled peach halves, torn burrata cheese, and toasted walnuts.
4. Drizzle with balsamic glaze and olive oil, and season with salt and pepper.
5. Gently toss to combine and serve immediately.

Nutritional Value: High in healthy fats, fiber, and various vitamins and minerals.

Food Class: Gluten-free, vegetarian.

Mediterranean Chickpea Salad

Prep Time: 15 minutes Serving Size: 4

Ingredients:

- 1 (15 oz) can chickpeas, rinsed and drained
- 1 cucumber, diced
- 1 red bell pepper, diced
- 1/2 red onion, diced
- 1/2 cup kalamata olives, pitted and halved
- 1/4 cup crumbled feta cheese
- 2 tablespoons olive oil
- 2 tablespoons lemon juice
- 2 tablespoons chopped fresh parsley
- Salt and pepper, to taste

Directions:

1. In a large bowl, combine the chickpeas, cucumber, bell pepper, red onion, olives, and feta cheese.
2. In a small bowl, whisk together the olive oil, lemon juice, parsley, and salt and pepper.
3. Pour the dressing over the chickpea mixture and toss to combine.
4. Serve chilled or at room temperature.

Nutritional Value: High in plant-based protein, fiber, healthy fats, and various vitamins and minerals.

Food Class: Gluten-free, vegetarian.

Salmon and Avocado Poke Bowl

Prep Time: 20 minutes Serving Size: 4

Ingredients:

- 1 lb. sushi-grade salmon, diced
- 1 avocado, diced
- 1 cup cooked brown rice
- 1 cup diced mango
- 1/4 cup diced red onion
- 2 tablespoons sesame seeds
- 2 tablespoons rice vinegar
- 2 tablespoons soy sauce (or tamari for gluten-free)
- 1 teaspoon sesame oil
- Salt and pepper, to taste

Directions:

1. In a large bowl, combine the diced salmon, avocado, cooked brown rice, mango, and red onion.
2. In a small bowl, whisk together the rice vinegar, soy sauce (or tamari), sesame oil, and a pinch of salt and pepper.
3. Pour the dressing over the salmon mixture and gently toss to combine.
4. Sprinkle with sesame seeds before serving.

Nutritional Value: High in healthy fats, protein, fiber, and various vitamins and minerals.

Food Class: Gluten-free (with tamari), can be made vegan by omitting the salmon.

Roasted Beet and Goat Cheese Salad

**Prep Time: 15 minutes Cook Time: 45 minutes
Serving Size: 4**

Ingredients:

- 4 medium beets, peeled and quartered
- 2 tablespoons olive oil
- Salt and pepper, to taste
- 4 cups mixed greens
- 1/4 cup crumbled goat cheese
- 1/4 cup toasted pecans
- 2 tablespoons balsamic vinegar

Directions:

1. Preheat the oven to 400°F (200°C).
2. Toss the quartered beets with olive oil, salt, and pepper, and arrange them on a baking sheet.
3. Roast for 40-45 minutes, or until the beets are tender and caramelized.
4. Let the roasted beets cool slightly, then slice or dice them.
5. In a large bowl, combine the mixed greens, roasted beets, crumbled goat cheese, and toasted pecans.
6. Drizzle with balsamic vinegar and toss to combine.

Nutritional Value: High in healthy fats, fiber, and various vitamins and minerals.

Food Class: Gluten-free, vegetarian.

Tropical Shrimp Salad

Prep Time: 20 minutes Serving Size: 4

Ingredients:

- 1 lb. cooked shrimp, peeled and deveined
- 1 cup diced mango
- 1 cup diced pineapple
- 1/4 cup diced red onion
- 1/4 cup chopped fresh cilantro
- 2 tablespoons lime juice
- 2 tablespoons olive oil
- Salt and pepper, to taste
- 4 cups mixed greens

Directions:

1. In a large bowl, combine the cooked shrimp, mango, pineapple, red onion, and cilantro.
2. In a small bowl, whisk together the lime juice, olive oil, and salt and pepper.
3. Pour the dressing over the shrimp mixture and gently toss to combine.
4. Serve the shrimp salad over mixed greens.

Nutritional Value: High in protein, healthy fats, fiber, and various vitamins and minerals.

Tuna Avocado Stuffed Tomatoes

Prep Time: 15 minutes Serving Size: 4

Ingredients:

- 4 large tomatoes
- 1 (5 oz) can tuna, drained
- 1 avocado, diced
- 2 tablespoons diced red onion
- 2 tablespoons lemon juice
- 2 tablespoons olive oil
- Salt and pepper, to taste
- Chopped parsley for garnish

Directions:

1. Cut the tops off the tomatoes and scoop out the insides, leaving a hollow tomato cup.
2. In a bowl, mix together the tuna, avocado, red onion, lemon juice, olive oil, salt, and pepper.
3. Spoon the tuna avocado mixture into the hollowed tomatoes.
4. Garnish with chopped parsley before serving.

Nutritional Value: High in protein, healthy fats, fiber, and various vitamins and minerals.

Food Class: Gluten-free, can be made vegan by omitting tuna and using mashed chickpeas instead.

Walnut Crusted Salmon Salad

**Prep Time: 15 minutes Cook Time: 12 minutes
Serving Size: 4**

Ingredients:

- 4 (6 oz) salmon fillets
- 1/2 cup walnuts, finely chopped
- 2 tablespoons Dijon mustard
- Salt and pepper, to taste
- 4 cups mixed greens
- 1 avocado, diced
- 2 tablespoons olive oil
- 2 tablespoons lemon juice

Directions:

1. Preheat oven to 400°F (200°C).
2. Pat the salmon fillets dry and season with salt and pepper.
3. Brush the top of each fillet with Dijon mustard and press the chopped walnuts onto the mustard to form a crust.
4. Bake for 10-12 minutes, or until salmon is cooked through.
5. In a large bowl, toss together the mixed greens, diced avocado, olive oil, and lemon juice.
6. Top the salad with the walnut-crusted salmon fillets.

Nutritional Value: High in protein, healthy fats, fiber, and various vitamins and minerals.

Food Class: Gluten-free.

Chicken Avocado Boats

Prep Time: 15 minutes Serving Size: 4

Ingredients:

- 2 avocados, halved and pitted
- 2 cups cooked shredded chicken
- 1/4 cup diced tomatoes
- 2 tablespoons diced red onion
- 2 tablespoons chopped fresh cilantro
- 2 tablespoons lime juice
- 1 tablespoon olive oil
- Salt and pepper, to taste

Directions:

1. Scoop out a little bit of the avocado flesh to create a larger cavity in each avocado half.
2. In a bowl, mix together the shredded chicken, tomatoes, red onion, cilantro, lime juice, olive oil, salt, and pepper.
3. Spoon the chicken mixture into the avocado halves.
4. Serve chilled or at room temperature.

Nutritional Value: High in protein, healthy fats, fiber, and various vitamins and minerals.

Food Class: Gluten-free, can be made vegan by using shredded jackfruit instead of chicken.

Salmon Niçoise Salad

Prep Time: 20 minutes Serving Size: 4

Ingredients:

- 4 (6 oz) salmon fillets
- 8 cups mixed greens
- 1 cup steamed green beans
- 1 cup cherry tomatoes, halved
- 1/2 cup Niçoise olives
- 2 hard-boiled eggs, quartered
- 2 tablespoons olive oil
- 2 tablespoons lemon juice
- 1 tablespoon Dijon mustard
- Salt and pepper, to taste

Directions:

1. Cook the salmon fillets by grilling, baking, or pan-searing until cooked through. Flake into bite-sized pieces.
2. In a large bowl, combine the mixed greens, green beans, cherry tomatoes, olives, and hard-boiled egg quarters.
3. In a small bowl, whisk together the olive oil, lemon juice, Dijon mustard, salt, and pepper to make the dressing.
4. Add the flaked salmon and dressing to the salad and toss gently to combine.

Nutritional Value: High in protein, healthy fats, fiber, and various vitamins and minerals.

Food Class: Gluten-free.

Avocado Tuna Lettuce Wraps

Prep Time: 15 minutes Serving Size: 4

Ingredients:

- 2 (5 oz) cans tuna, drained
- 1 avocado, diced
- 1/4 cup diced red onion
- 2 tablespoons lemon juice
- 2 tablespoons olive oil
- Salt and pepper, to taste
- 8 large lettuce leaves

Directions:

1. In a bowl, mix together the tuna, avocado, red onion, lemon juice, olive oil, salt, and pepper.
2. Spoon the tuna avocado mixture into the lettuce leaves, dividing it evenly.
3. Serve chilled or at room temperature.

Nutritional Value: High in protein, healthy fats, fiber, and various vitamins and minerals.

Food Class: Gluten-free, can be made vegan by using mashed chickpeas instead of tuna.

Nutty Crunch Salad

Prep Time: 15 minutes Serving Size: 4

Ingredients:

- 4 cups mixed greens
- 1 cup sliced strawberries
- 1/4 cup sliced almonds
- 1/4 cup pecan halves
- 1/4 cup crumbled feta cheese (optional)
- 2 tablespoons olive oil
- 2 tablespoons balsamic vinegar
- Salt and pepper, to taste

Directions:

1. In a large bowl, combine the mixed greens, sliced strawberries, almonds, pecans, and feta cheese (if using).
2. In a small bowl, whisk together the olive oil, balsamic vinegar, salt, and pepper to make the dressing.
3. Pour the dressing over the salad and toss gently to combine.

Nutritional Value: High in healthy fats, fiber, and various vitamins and minerals.

Food Class: Gluten-free, can be made vegan by omitting the feta cheese.

Chapter 8: Dinners

Dinner Entrees and One-Dish Meals

Highlighting Good Fats

Avocado Stuffed Chicken Breasts

**Prep Time: 15 minutes Cook Time: 25 minutes
Serving Size: 4**

Ingredients:

- 4 boneless, skinless chicken breasts
- 2 ripe avocados, pitted and mashed
- 1/2 cup shredded cheddar cheese (or dairy-free alternative)
- 1/4 cup breadcrumbs (or gluten-free breadcrumbs)
- 2 tablespoons olive oil
- Salt and pepper, to taste

Directions:

1. Preheat the oven to 375°F (190°C).
2. Pound the chicken breasts to an even thickness and season with salt and pepper.
3. In a bowl, combine the mashed avocado and shredded cheese.
4. Stuff the chicken breasts with the avocado-cheese mixture and secure with toothpicks if needed.
5. Coat the stuffed chicken with breadcrumbs and place in a baking dish.
6. Drizzle with olive oil and bake for 25-30 minutes, or until the chicken is cooked through.

Nutritional Value: High in protein, healthy fats, and various vitamins and minerals.

Food Class: Gluten-free (with gluten-free breadcrumbs), can be made dairy-free (with dairy-free cheese alternative).

Lentil and Sweet Potato Buddha Bowls

**Prep Time: 15 minutes Cook Time: 30 minutes
Serving Size: 4**

Ingredients:

- 1 cup dried lentils
- 2 medium sweet potatoes, diced
- 1 avocado, diced
- 1/4 cup toasted pumpkin seeds
- 4 cups baby spinach or mixed greens
- 2 tablespoons olive oil
- 2 tablespoons lemon juice
- Salt and pepper, to taste

Directions:

1. Cook the lentils according to package instructions and set aside.
2. Preheat the oven to 400°F (200°C).
3. Toss the diced sweet potatoes with olive oil, salt, and pepper, and spread them on a baking sheet.
4. Roast the sweet potatoes for 25-30 minutes, or until tender and caramelized.
5. In a large bowl, combine the cooked lentils, roasted sweet potatoes, avocado, pumpkin seeds, and greens.
6. Drizzle with lemon juice and toss gently to combine.

Nutritional Value: High in fiber, plant-based protein, healthy fats, and various vitamins and minerals.

Food Class: Vegan, gluten-free.

Salmon with Creamy Dill Sauce

**Prep Time: 10 minutes Cook Time: 15 minutes
Serving Size: 4**

Ingredients:

- 4 (6 oz) salmon fillets
- 1/2 cup Greek yogurt (or plant-based yogurt alternative)
- 1/4 cup chopped fresh dill
- 2 tablespoons lemon juice
- 2 tablespoons olive oil
- Salt and pepper, to taste

Directions:

1. Preheat the oven to 400°F (200°C).
2. In a small bowl, mix together the Greek yogurt, dill, lemon juice, and a pinch of salt and pepper to make the dill sauce.
3. Place the salmon fillets on a baking sheet lined with parchment paper or a silicone mat.
4. Drizzle the salmon with olive oil and season with salt and pepper.
5. Bake for 12-15 minutes, or until the salmon is cooked through.
6. Serve the salmon fillets with the creamy dill sauce on the side.

Nutritional Value: High in protein, healthy fats, and various vitamins and minerals.

Beef and Vegetable Stir-Fry with Cashews

**Prep Time: 15 minutes Cook Time: 20 minutes
Serving Size: 4**

Ingredients:

- 1 lb. sirloin steak, thinly sliced
- 2 tablespoons coconut oil (or avocado oil)
- 1 red bell pepper, sliced
- 1 cup broccoli florets
- 1 cup sliced mushrooms
- 1/2 cup roasted cashews
- 2 tablespoons soy sauce (or tamari for gluten-free)
- 2 tablespoons rice vinegar
- 1 teaspoon sesame oil
- Salt and pepper, to taste

Directions:

1. In a large skillet or wok, heat the coconut oil over high heat.
2. Add the sliced steak and stir-fry until browned and nearly cooked through, about 5 minutes.
3. Add the bell pepper, broccoli, and mushrooms to the skillet and continue to stir-fry for another 5-7 minutes, or until the vegetables are tender-crisp.
4. In a small bowl, whisk together the soy sauce (or tamari), rice vinegar, sesame oil, and a pinch of salt and pepper.
5. Pour the sauce over the stir-fry and toss to combine.
6. Remove from heat and stir in the roasted cashews.
7. Serve over steamed rice or cauliflower rice, if desired.

Nutritional Value: High in protein, healthy fats, and various vitamins and minerals.

Food Class: Gluten-free (with tamari), dairy-free.

Baked Cod with Almond-Herb Crust

**Prep Time: 15 minutes Cook Time: 20 minutes
Serving Size: 4**

Ingredients:

- 4 (6 oz) cod fillets
- 1/2 cup almond flour
- 1/4 cup grated Parmesan cheese (or dairy-free alternative)
- 2 tablespoons chopped fresh parsley
- 2 tablespoons olive oil
- 1 lemon, sliced into wedges

Directions:

1. Preheat the oven to 400°F (200°C).
2. In a shallow bowl, mix together the almond flour, Parmesan cheese (or dairy-free alternative), and chopped parsley.
3. Brush the cod fillets with olive oil and dip them into the almond-herb mixture, coating both sides.
4. Place the coated cod fillets on a baking sheet lined with parchment paper or a silicone mat.
5. Bake for 18-20 minutes, or until the fish flakes easily with a fork.
6. Serve the baked cod with lemon wedges on the side.

Nutritional Value: High in protein, healthy fats, and various vitamins and minerals.

Food Class: Gluten-free, can be made dairy-free (with dairy-free Parmesan alternative).

Vegetable Frittata with Goat Cheese

**Prep Time: 15 minutes Cook Time: 20 minutes
Serving Size: 4**

Ingredients:

- 8 eggs
- 1/4 cup milk (or plant-based milk alternative)
- 1 cup diced bell peppers
- 1 cup sliced mushrooms
- 1/2 cup diced onion
- 1/2 cup crumbled goat cheese (or dairy-free alternative)
- 2 tablespoons olive oil
- Salt and pepper, to taste

Directions:

1. Preheat the oven to 350°F (175°C).
2. In a large bowl, whisk together the eggs and milk (or plant-based milk alternative). Season with salt and pepper.
3. In an oven-safe skillet, heat the olive oil over medium heat.
4. Add the bell peppers, mushrooms, and onion to the skillet and sauté for 5 minutes, or until softened.
5. Pour the egg mixture over the sautéed vegetables and sprinkle with the crumbled goat cheese (or dairy-free alternative).
6. Transfer the skillet to the oven and bake for 15-20 minutes, or until the frittata is set and golden brown on top.
7. Let cool for 5 minutes before slicing and serving.

Greek Lamb Meatballs with Tzatziki Sauce

**Prep Time: 20 minutes Cook Time: 20 minutes
Serving Size: 4**

Ingredients:

For the meatballs:

- 1 lb. ground lamb
- 1 egg
- 1/2 cup breadcrumbs (or gluten-free breadcrumbs)
- 1/4 cup crumbled feta cheese
- 2 tablespoons chopped fresh parsley
- 1 teaspoon dried oregano
- Salt and pepper, to taste
- 2 tablespoons olive oil

For the tzatziki sauce:

- 1 cup Greek yogurt (or plant-based yogurt alternative)
- 1/2 cucumber, grated and drained
- 2 tablespoons lemon juice
- 1 clove garlic, minced
- 2 tablespoons chopped fresh dill
- Salt and pepper, to taste

Directions:

1. Preheat the oven to 400°F (200°C).
2. In a large bowl, combine the ground lamb, egg, breadcrumbs, feta cheese, parsley, oregano, salt, and pepper. Mix well until fully incorporated.
3. Form the mixture into 1-inch meatballs and place them on a baking sheet lined with parchment paper or a silicone mat.
4. Drizzle the meatballs with olive oil and bake for 18-20 minutes, or until cooked through.
5. While the meatballs are baking, prepare the tzatziki sauce by mixing together the yogurt, grated cucumber, lemon juice, garlic, dill, salt, and pepper.
6. Serve the warm meatballs with the tzatziki sauce on the side.

Nutritional Value: High in protein, healthy fats, and various vitamins and minerals.

Food Class: Gluten-free (with gluten-free breadcrumbs), can be made dairy-free (with plant-based yogurt and omitting feta cheese).

Maple Walnut Crusted Salmon

**Prep Time: 15 minutes Cook Time: 15 minutes
Serving Size: 4**

Ingredients:

- 4 (6 oz) salmon fillets
- 1/2 cup walnuts, finely chopped
- 2 tablespoons maple syrup
- 2 tablespoons Dijon mustard
- Salt and pepper, to taste
- 2 tablespoons olive oil

Directions:

1. Preheat the oven to 400°F (200°C).
2. In a shallow bowl, mix together the chopped walnuts, maple syrup, and Dijon mustard. Season with salt and pepper.
3. Brush the salmon fillets with olive oil and then dip them into the walnut-maple mixture, coating both sides.
4. Place the coated salmon fillets on a baking sheet lined with parchment paper or a silicone mat.
5. Bake for 12-15 minutes, or until the salmon is cooked through and the crust is golden brown.

Nutritional Value: High in protein, healthy fats, and various vitamins and minerals.

Food Class: Gluten-free.

Shrimp Scampi with Zoodles

Prep Time: 15 minutes Cook Time: 15 minutes

Serving Size: 4

Ingredients:

- 1 lb. shrimp, peeled and deveined
- 4 zucchinis, spiralized into noodles
- 4 cloves garlic, minced
- 2 tablespoons lemon juice
- 1/4 cup white wine (or chicken broth for non-alcoholic option)
- 1/4 cup olive oil
- 2 tablespoons butter (or plant-based butter alternative)
- 1/4 cup grated Parmesan cheese (or dairy-free alternative)
- 2 tablespoons chopped fresh parsley
- Salt and pepper, to taste

Directions:

1. In a large skillet, heat the olive oil and butter (or plant-based butter alternative) over medium-high heat.
2. Add the minced garlic and sauté for 1 minute, being careful not to burn it.
3. Add the shrimp and cook for 2-3 minutes, or until they start to turn pink.
4. Add the white wine (or chicken broth) and lemon juice, and simmer for 2-3 minutes.
5. Add the zucchini noodles and toss everything together with tongs or a wooden spoon.
6. Cook for an additional 2-3 minutes, or until the zucchini noodles are tender but still crisp.

7. Remove from heat and stir in the grated Parmesan cheese (or dairy-free alternative) and chopped parsley.
8. Season with salt and pepper to taste.

Nutritional Value: High in protein, healthy fats, and various vitamins and minerals.

Food Class: Gluten-free, can be made dairy-free (with plant-based butter and cheese alternatives).

Coconut Chicken Curry

**Prep Time: 15 minutes Cook Time: 30 minutes
Serving Size: 4**

Ingredients:

- 1 lb. boneless, skinless chicken breasts, cut into 1-inch pieces
- 1 (13.5 oz) can coconut milk
- 1 cup chicken broth
- 2 tablespoons red curry paste
- 2 tablespoons coconut oil
- 1 onion, diced
- 3 cloves garlic, minced
- 1 tablespoon grated fresh ginger
- 1 bell pepper, sliced
- 1 cup sliced mushrooms
- 2 tablespoons lime juice
- Salt and pepper, to taste
- Chopped fresh cilantro for garnish

Directions:

1. In a large skillet or Dutch oven, heat the coconut oil over medium heat.
2. Add the diced onion and sauté for 2-3 minutes, or until softened.
3. Add the minced garlic and grated ginger, and cook for 1 minute more.
4. Add the red curry paste and stir to combine.
5. Pour in the coconut milk and chicken broth, and whisk to incorporate the curry paste.
6. Add the chicken pieces, bell pepper, and mushrooms to the skillet. Season with salt and pepper.

7. Bring the mixture to a simmer and cook for 15-20 minutes, or until the chicken is cooked through and the vegetables are tender.
8. Stir in the lime juice and garnish with chopped fresh cilantro.
9. Serve over steamed rice or cauliflower rice.

Nutritional Value: High in protein, healthy fats, and various vitamins and minerals from the chicken, coconut milk, vegetables, and spices.

Food Class: Gluten-free, dairy-free.

Tips for Modifying Recipes for Dietary

Restrictions

1. Gluten-Free: When modifying recipes for a gluten-free diet, substitute wheat flour with gluten-free alternatives like almond flour, coconut flour, or gluten-free all-purpose flour. Use gluten-free breadcrumbs or crushed nuts for coating or binding. Choose gluten-free tamari or coconut aminos instead of soy sauce.

2. Dairy-Free: To make recipes dairy-free, replace milk with plant-based alternatives like almond milk, coconut milk, or oat milk. Use dairy-free cheese alternatives or omit cheese altogether. Substitute butter with olive oil, coconut oil, or plant-based butter substitutes.

3. Vegan: For vegan modifications, omit all animal-based products like meat, fish, eggs, and dairy. Replace these with plant-based protein sources like tofu, tempeh, lentils, or plant-based meat alternatives. Use plant-based milk, cheese, and butter substitutes as needed.

4. Nut-Free: If catering to nut allergies, replace nuts and nut-based ingredients with seeds (like pumpkin, sunflower, or sesame seeds) or swap them with other crunchy ingredients like breadcrumbs or crushed crackers.

5. Vegetarian: To make recipes vegetarian-friendly, simply omit any meat or fish ingredients and replace them with plant-based protein sources like beans, lentils, tofu, or vegetarian meat alternatives.

6. Low-Carb/Keto: For low-carb or keto diets, replace high-carb ingredients like rice, pasta, and breadcrumbs with low-carb alternatives like cauliflower rice, zucchini noodles, or almond flour. Increase the portions of healthy fats like olive oil, avocado, and nuts/seeds.

7. Read Labels: Always read ingredient labels carefully when purchasing pre-made or packaged products to ensure they align with your dietary restrictions.

8. Experiment and Adjust: Don't be afraid to experiment with ingredient substitutions and adjust seasoning and cooking times as needed when modifying recipes. Start with small changes and adjust to your preferences.

Chapter 9: Snacks & Treats

Nutrient-dense, High-Fat Snack Ideas

Mixed Nuts Trail Mix

Prep Time: 10 minutes Serving Size: 8

Ingredients:

- 1 cup almonds
- 1 cup cashews
- 1/2 cup walnuts
- 1/2 cup pecans
- 1/4 cup pumpkin seeds
- 1/4 cup dried cranberries
- 2 tablespoons coconut flakes
- 1 tablespoon chia seeds
- 1 tablespoon honey (optional)
- 1/2 teaspoon ground cinnamon
- 1/4 teaspoon sea salt

Directions:

1. In a large bowl, combine the almonds, cashews, walnuts, pecans, pumpkin seeds, dried cranberries, coconut flakes, and chia seeds.
2. If using honey, drizzle it over the nut mixture and toss to coat.
3. Sprinkle the cinnamon and sea salt over the trail mix and toss again to evenly distribute.
4. Store in an airtight container for up to 2 weeks.

Nutritional Value: High in healthy fats, fiber, protein, and various vitamins and minerals.

Food Class: Vegan, gluten-free.

Avocado Brownies

**Prep Time: 15 minutes Cook Time: 25 minutes
Serving Size: 12**

Ingredients:

- 1 ripe avocado, mashed
- 1/2 cup coconut sugar
- 1/2 cup unsweetened cocoa powder
- 2 eggs (or flax eggs for vegan)
- 1 teaspoon vanilla extract
- 1/2 cup almond flour
- 1/2 teaspoon baking soda
- 1/4 teaspoon sea salt
- 1/2 cup dark chocolate chips (or dairy-free chocolate chips)

Directions:

1. Preheat the oven to 350°F (175°C). Grease an 8x8-inch baking pan.
2. In a large bowl, combine the mashed avocado, coconut sugar, cocoa powder, eggs (or flax eggs), and vanilla extract. Mix well until smooth.
3. Add the almond flour, baking soda, and sea salt to the wet ingredients and stir until fully incorporated.
4. Fold in the dark chocolate chips.
5. Pour the brownie batter into the prepared baking pan and smooth the top with a spatula.
6. Bake for 20-25 minutes, or until a toothpick inserted in the center comes out clean.
7. Allow the brownies to cool completely before cutting into squares.

Nutritional Value: High in healthy fats, fiber, and various vitamins and minerals.

Food Class: Gluten-free, can be made vegan (with flax eggs and dairy-free chocolate chips).

Coconut Energy Bites

Prep Time: 10 minutes Serving Size: 12

Ingredients:

- 1 cup rolled oats
- 1/2 cup shredded coconut
- 1/2 cup almond butter
- 1/4 cup honey
- 1/4 cup ground flaxseed
- 1/4 cup mini chocolate chips (or dairy-free chocolate chips)
- 1 teaspoon vanilla extract
- 1/4 teaspoon sea salt

Directions:

1. In a large bowl, mix together the rolled oats, shredded coconut, almond butter, honey, ground flaxseed, mini chocolate chips, vanilla extract, and sea salt until well combined.
2. Using your hands, roll the mixture into small balls, about 1-inch in size.
3. Store the energy bites in an airtight container in the refrigerator for up to 2 weeks.

Nutritional Value: High in healthy fats, fiber, protein, and various vitamins and minerals.

Food Class: Gluten-free, can be made vegan (with maple syrup or agave nectar instead of honey and dairy-free chocolate chips).

Decadent but Healthy Dessert Recipes

Chocolate Avocado Mousse

Prep Time: 10 minutes Serving Size: 4

Ingredients:

- 2 ripe avocados, pitted and mashed
- 1/2 cup unsweetened cocoa powder
- 1/4 cup maple syrup
- 1/4 cup unsweetened almond milk
- 1 teaspoon vanilla extract
- 1/4 teaspoon sea salt
- Coconut whipped cream (optional)
- Berries for garnish (optional)

1. Directions:
2. In a food processor or blender, combine the mashed avocados, cocoa powder, maple syrup, almond milk, vanilla extract, and sea salt. Process until smooth and creamy.
3. Spoon the mousse into individual serving bowls or glasses.
4. If desired, top with coconut whipped cream and fresh berries.
5. Refrigerate until ready to serve.

Nutritional Value: High in healthy fats, fiber, and various vitamins and minerals.

Food Class: Vegan, gluten-free.

Coconut Chia Pudding

Prep Time: 5 minutes (plus overnight soaking)
Serving Size: 4

Ingredients:

- 1 cup unsweetened coconut milk
- 1/2 cup chia seeds
- 2 tablespoons maple syrup
- 1 teaspoon vanilla extract
- 1/2 cup fresh or frozen mango, diced
- 2 tablespoons shredded coconut

Directions:

1. In a jar or bowl, combine the coconut milk, chia seeds, maple syrup, and vanilla extract. Stir well.
2. Cover and refrigerate overnight (or for at least 4 hours) to allow the chia seeds to swell and form a pudding-like consistency.
3. Before serving, stir in the diced mango and shredded coconut.

Nutritional Value: High in healthy fats, fiber, and various vitamins and minerals.

Food Class: Vegan, gluten-free.

Almond Butter Cups

Prep Time: 15 minutes Serving Size: 12

Ingredients:

- 1 cup almond butter
- 1/4 cup coconut oil, melted
- 1/4 cup maple syrup
- 1 teaspoon vanilla extract
- 1/4 teaspoon sea salt
- 1 cup dark chocolate chips (or dairy-free chocolate chips)
- 1 tablespoon coconut oil (for melting the chocolate)

Directions:

1. In a bowl, mix together the almond butter, melted coconut oil, maple syrup, vanilla extract, and sea salt until well combined.
2. Line a muffin tin with cupcake liners.
3. Divide the almond butter mixture evenly among the lined muffin cups, pressing it down to create a flat surface.
4. In a double boiler or microwave-safe bowl, melt the dark chocolate chips with the remaining 1 tablespoon of coconut oil, stirring until smooth.
5. Spoon the melted chocolate over the almond butter cups, covering the tops.
6. Refrigerate for at least 2 hours, or until the chocolate has hardened.

Nutritional Value: High in healthy fats, protein, and various vitamins and minerals.

Food Class: Gluten-free, can be made vegan (with dairy-free chocolate chips).

Chapter 10: Tips & Tricks

Stocking a Healthy Menopause Kitchen

During menopause, it's essential to have a well-stocked kitchen that supports your nutritional needs and overall wellness. Here are some valuable tips for stocking your menopause kitchen:

1. Focus on Healthy Fats: Make sure to have a variety of healthy fats on hand, such as avocados, olive oil, nuts (almonds, walnuts, pecans), seeds (chia, flaxseed, pumpkin), fatty fish (salmon, mackerel, sardines), and nut butters. These fats can help manage hot flashes, support hormone balance, and promote heart health.

2. Stock Up on Lean Proteins: Lean proteins like chicken, turkey, eggs, tofu, tempeh, and legumes are crucial for maintaining muscle mass, which can decline during menopause. They also help regulate blood sugar levels and keep you feeling fuller for longer.

3. Embrace Whole Grains: opt for whole grains like quinoa, brown rice, oats, and whole-wheat pasta, which provide fiber, B vitamins, and other essential nutrients. Fiber can help alleviate constipation, a common issue during menopause.

4. Load Up on Fruits and Veggies: Fresh, frozen, or canned fruits and vegetables should be a staple in your menopause kitchen. They're packed with antioxidants, vitamins, and minerals that support overall health and may help reduce menopause symptoms like hot flashes and mood swings.

5. Keep Flavorful Herbs and Spices: Stock up on fresh and dried herbs and spices like turmeric, ginger, cinnamon, and cayenne pepper. They not only add flavor to your dishes but also offer anti-inflammatory and antioxidant properties.

6. Have Plant-Based Milks: Keep a variety of plant-based milks on hand, such as almond, coconut, or oat milk, as they're rich in vitamins and minerals and can be a great alternative for those with lactose intolerance, which can develop during menopause.

7. Don't Forget Probiotics: Incorporate probiotic-rich foods like yogurt, kefir, sauerkraut, and kombucha into your diet. Probiotics can help support gut health, which is crucial for hormone balance and overall well-being.

8. Stay Hydrated: Keep plenty of water, herbal teas, and infused waters on hand to stay hydrated, which can help alleviate menopause symptoms like hot flashes and mood swings.

By stocking your menopause kitchen with these essential items, you'll have everything you need to create delicious, nutrient-dense meals and snacks that support your body's changing needs during this transition.

Shopping Lists for Good Fat Essentials

To make grocery shopping a breeze and ensure you always have a well-stocked menopause kitchen, here are some handy shopping lists for good fat essentials:

Oils and Condiments

- Extra virgin olive oil
- Avocado oil
- Coconut oil
- Nut oils (walnut, almond, hazelnut)
- Tahini (sesame seed paste)
- Nut butters (almond, peanut, cashew)
- Olives and olive tapenade
- Pesto
- Hummus

Nuts and Seeds

- Almonds
- Walnuts
- Pecans
- Cashews
- Pistachios
- Chia seeds
- Flaxseeds
- Pumpkin seeds
- Sunflower seeds

Fruits and Vegetables

- Avocados
- Olives
- Coconuts
- Leafy greens (spinach, kale, arugula)
- Berries (blueberries, raspberries, strawberries)
- Tomatoes
- Bell peppers
- Cucumber
- Carrots
- Broccoli
- Sweet potatoes

Dairy and Alternatives

- Greek yogurt
- Cottage cheese
- Feta cheese
- Almond milk
- Coconut milk
- Oat milk

Seafood

- Salmon
- Sardines
- Mackerel
- Tuna
- Shrimp

Pantry Staples

- Canned coconut milk
- Nut flours (almond, coconut)
- Chia seeds
- Flaxseeds
- Dark chocolate (at least 70% cacao)
- Cocoa powder
- Coconut flakes

By keeping these good fat essentials well-stocked in your kitchen, you'll have the building blocks for creating delicious, nutrient-dense meals and snacks that support your overall health and well-being during menopause.

Simple Exercises and Self-Care Practices for Menopause

Dear reader, as you navigate the journey of menopause, it's crucial to prioritize not only your nutritional needs but also your overall well-being. Incorporating simple exercises and self-care practices into your routine can greatly alleviate the physical and emotional challenges that often accompany this transitional phase. Let's explore some valuable strategies that can help you feel your best during this time.

Exercise is a powerful tool for managing menopause symptoms and supporting your overall health. Regular physical activity can help alleviate hot flashes, improve sleep quality, boost mood, and maintain bone density – all common concerns during menopause. Here are some simple yet effective exercises to consider:

1. Walking: This low-impact activity is accessible to most people and can be easily incorporated into your daily routine. Aim for at least 30 minutes of brisk walking each day, or break it up into shorter intervals if needed. Walking not only supports cardiovascular health but also provides an opportunity to enjoy the outdoors and clear your mind.

2. Strength Training: Resistance exercises are essential for building and maintaining muscle mass, which can decrease during menopause. Incorporate exercises like squats, lunges, and weightlifting into your routine. You can use your body weight, resistance bands, or light dumbbells. Strength training also helps to improve bone density and reduce the risk of osteoporosis.

3. Yoga and Pilates: These mind-body practices combine gentle stretching, strengthening, and breathing techniques. They can help reduce stress, improve flexibility, and promote a sense of calm and relaxation. Look for beginner-friendly classes or follow online tutorials to learn the basics.

4. Swimming or Water Aerobics: Low-impact water exercises are an excellent option for those experiencing joint pain or discomfort during menopause. The buoyancy of the water reduces stress on the joints while providing resistance for strength training and cardiovascular conditioning.

Remember, it's essential to start slowly and gradually increase the intensity and duration of your exercises. Listen to your body and adjust your routine as needed. Consult with a healthcare professional or certified fitness instructor, especially if you have any underlying health conditions or concerns.

In addition to regular exercise, self-care practices can play a significant role in managing menopause symptoms and promoting overall well-being. Here are some self-care strategies to consider:

1. Stress Management: Menopause can be a stressful time, both physically and emotionally. Incorporate stress-reducing activities into your daily routine, such as deep breathing exercises, meditation, journaling, or practicing mindfulness. These practices can help lower cortisol levels, reduce anxiety, and improve overall mood.

2. Sleep Hygiene: Hot flashes, night sweats, and hormonal fluctuations can disrupt sleep patterns during menopause. Establish a consistent sleep routine by going to bed and waking up at the same time each day. Create a cool, dark, and comfortable sleep environment, and avoid consuming caffeine or engaging in stimulating activities close to bedtime.

3. Relaxation Techniques: Explore techniques like progressive muscle relaxation, guided imagery, or aromatherapy to promote a sense of calm and relaxation. These practices can help counteract the stress and anxiety that often accompany menopause symptoms.

4. Social Support: Surround yourself with a supportive network of friends, family, or a menopause support group. Sharing your experiences and concerns with others going through similar situations can provide valuable insights, emotional support, and a sense of community.

5. Mind-Body Connection: Practices like yoga, tai chi, or qigong can help cultivate a mind-body connection, reducing stress and promoting a sense of balance and well-being. These gentle movements can also improve flexibility, balance, and overall physical health.

6. Pampering and Self-Care: Treat yourself to activities that bring you joy and relaxation, such as taking a warm bath, getting a massage, reading a good book, or engaging in a creative hobby. These simple pleasures can help boost your mood and provide a much-needed break from the stresses of daily life.

Always put at the back of your mind that menopause is a natural transition, and every woman's experience is unique. It's essential to listen to your body, be patient with yourself, and make adjustments as needed. Don't hesitate to seek support from healthcare professionals, counselors, or support groups if you're struggling with menopause symptoms or related concerns.

CONCLUSION

Here we are at the final pages of this book, I hope you have gained a deeper understanding of the profound impact that good fats can have on your overall well-being, particularly during the challenging transition of menopause. The recipes we have explored together are not merely a collection of tasty dishes; they represent a holistic approach to nourishing your body, mind, and spirit.

Throughout this journey, we have delved into the intricate world of good fats, uncovering their numerous benefits, from promoting hormonal balance and reducing inflammation to supporting cognitive function and cardiovascular health. By incorporating these nutrient-dense ingredients into your daily meals, you are taking a proactive step towards embracing the changes that come with menopause, empowering yourself to thrive during this transformative phase of life.

I want to emphasize the importance of embracing this lifestyle change with patience and self-compassion. Menopause is a unique experience for every woman, and there is no one-size-fits-all solution. However, by making conscious choices about the foods we consume, we can alleviate many of the common symptoms associated with this transition, such as hot flashes, mood swings, and weight fluctuations.

The recipes in this book are not mere placeholders; they are carefully crafted to provide you with a delightful culinary experience while simultaneously nourishing your body with the essential nutrients it craves. From the vibrant salads bursting with flavor to the comforting and satisfying main dishes, each recipe is a testament to the power of good fats in creating balanced and delicious meals.

As we part ways, I encourage you to continue exploring the world of good fats and their countless benefits. Embrace this newfound knowledge as a lifelong companion, allowing it to guide you towards a path of vibrant health and well-being. Remember, small changes can have a profound impact, and every step you take towards a healthier lifestyle is a step closer to embracing the best version of yourself.

If you found this book insightful and the recipes enjoyable, I would be forever grateful if you could take a moment to leave a review. Your feedback not only helps me to improve and refine my work but also allows others to discover the transformative power of good fats in their own menopausal journey. Together, we can create a ripple effect, empowering women worldwide to embrace this pivotal phase of life with grace, vitality, and a renewed sense of well-being.

Thank you for joining me on this journey. May the knowledge you have gained from these pages serve as a guiding light, illuminating your path towards a healthier, more balanced, and fulfilling life.